OFFICE
HYSTEROSCOPY

OFFICE
HYSTEROSCOPY

Edited by

Keith B. Isaacson, M.D.

Chief, Vincent Memorial Endocrinology and Infertility Division
Massachusetts General Hospital
Assistant Professor of Obstetrics, Gynecology, and Reproductive Biology
Harvard Medical School
Boston, Massachusetts

with 151 illustrations

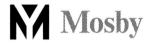 Mosby

St. Louis Baltimore Boston Carlsbad Chicago Naples New York Philadelphia Portland
London Madrid Mexico City Singapore Sydney Tokyo Toronto Wiesbaden

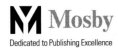

Dedicated to Publishing Excellence

A Times Mirror
Company

Publisher: Anne S. Patterson
Editor: Susie Baxter
Developmental Editor: Ellen Baker Geisel
Project Manager: Mark Spann
Production Editor: Anne Salmo
Designer: Judi Lang
Manufacturing Manager: Tony McAllister
Cover art: Edith Tagrin

Copyright © 1996 by Mosby-Year Book, Inc.

Printed in the United States of America

Composition by Graphic World, Inc.
Printed by Buxton Skinner Printing Co.

Mosby–Year Book, Inc.
11830 Westline Industrial Drive
St. Louis, Missouri 63146

Library of Congress Cataloging-in-Publication Data

Office hysteroscopy / edited by Keith B. Isaacson.
    p.   cm.
    Includes bibliographical references and index.
    ISBN 0-8151-4842-9
    1. Hysteroscopy.   2. Ambulatory medical care.   I. Isaacson, Keith
B.
    [DNLM: 1. Hysteroscopy—methods.   2. Ambulatory Care.   WP 440 032
1996]
RG304.5.H97034   1996
618.1'407545—dc20
DNLM/DLC
for Library of Congress   96-2065
                                                     CIP

96 97 98 99 00 / 9 8 7 6 5 4 3 2 1

CONTRIBUTORS

Johnny T. Awwad, M.D.
Clinical Instructor
Department of Obstetrics, Gynecology, and Reproductive
 Biology
Harvard School of Medicine
Clinical Fellow
Department of Reproductive Endocrinology and Infertility
Massachusetts General Hospital
Boston, Massachusetts

John D. Bertrand, M.D.
Clinical Professor
University of Texas Southwestern Medical School
Director, Reproductive Surgery
Presbyterian Hospital Dallas
Department of Obstetrics and Gynecology
Dallas, Texas

John R. Brumsted, M.D.
Associate Professor
Department of Obstetrics and Gynecology
University of Vermont College of Medicine
Director, Reproductive Endocrinology & Infertility
Head, Section of Gynecology
Department of Obstetrics and Gynecology
Fletcher Allen Health Care
Burlington, Vermont

Patricia A. Caplinger, M.D.
Clinical Professor
Department of Obstetrics & Gynecology
Phoenix Baptist Hospital
Good Samaritan Medical Center
Phoenix, Arizona

Jay M. Cooper, M.D.
Department of Obstretrics & Gynecology
Phoenix Baptist Hospital
Phoenix, Arizona

Alan H. DeCherney, M.D.
Louis E. Phaneuf Professor and Chairman
Department of Obstetrics and Gynecology
Tufts University School of Medicine and New England
 Medical Center
Boston, Massachusetts

Richard J. Gimpelson, M.D.
Assistant Clinical Professor
Department of Obstetrics & Gynecology
St. Louis University School of Medicine
St. Louis, Missouri

Keith B. Isaacson, M.D.
Chief, Vincent Memorial Endocrinology and Infertility
 Division
Massachusetts General Hospital
Assistant Professor of Obstetrics, Gynecology, and
 Reproductive Biology
Harvard Medical School
Boston, Massachusetts

Louise Lapensee, M.D.
Vincent Memorial Obstetrics and Gynecology Service
Harvard Medical School
Massachusetts General Hospital
Boston, Massachusetts

Franklin D. Loffer, M.D.
Director, Gynecologic Endoscopy
Department of Obstetrics and Gynecology
Maricopa Medical Center
Phoenix, Arizona

René Marty, M.D.
Spécialiste Gynécologue Obstétricien
Attaché Consultant
Department of Gynécologie
Centre Hospitalo-Universitaire et de Recherche
Responsable de Unité d'Hystéroscopie Flexible
Hopital Avicenne
Paris, France

Patricia Mussuto, M.D.
Faculty of Medecine
Broussais Hotel-Dieu
Attache Des Hospitaux
Paris, France

Misty Blanchette Porter, M.D.
Fellow, Reproductive Endocrinology and Infertility
Department of Obstetrics and Gynecology
Division of Reproductive Endocrinology and Infertility
University of Vermont College of Medicine
Clinical Instructor
Department of Obstetrics and Gynecology
Division of Reproductive Endocrinology and Infertility
Fletcher Allen Health Care
Burlington, Vermont

Maryse D. Roudier, M.P.H.
Department of Obstetrics and Gynecology
Tufts University School of Medicine and New England
  Medical Center
Boston, Massachusetts

Maureen P. Spencer, M.Ed., R.N., C.I.C.
Assistant Professor
Graduate Nursing Program
Institute of Health Professions
Director, Infection Control Unit
Massachusetts General Hospital
Boston, Massachusetts

Eric S. Surrey, M.D.
Medical Director
Center for Reproductive Medicine and Surgery
Beverly Hills, California
Associate Clinical Professor
Department of Obstetrics/Gynecology
UCLA School of Medicine
Los Angeles, California

Suzanne O. Tempesta, R.N., B.S.
Department of Gynecology
Massachusetts General Hospital
Boston, Massachusetts

Rafael F. Valle, M.D.
Professor of Obstetrics and Gynecology
Division of Reproductive Endocrinology and Infertility
Northwestern University Medical School
Attending Physician
Department of Obstetrics and Gynecology
Prentice Women's Hospital and Maternity Center of
  Northwestern Memorial Hospital
Chicago, Illinois

Kees Wamsteker, M.D., Ph.D.
Spaarne Hospital
Department of Obstetrics and Gynaecology
Van Heythuizenweg
Hysteroscopy Training Centre
Haarlem, The Netherlands

To my father, Herschel David Isaacson,
whose encouragement remains my inspiration.

FOREWORD

Hysteroscopy had been a dream for many years before becoming reality in the early 1980s. However, general acceptance of hysteroscopic techniques as part of the gynecologist's armamentarium was delayed until hysteroscopy could be used in operative procedures. The origin of hysteroscopy dates back to the primitive stages of endoscopy at the turn of the 20th century when the majority of endoscopic procedures were cystoscopic and laryngobronchoscopic. In the 1950s I.C. Rubin tried to modify the Rubin insufflator, which tested tubal patency, to function as a hysteroscope, but he was unable to generate enough pressure to separate the walls of the uterus—all he saw was a red, homogeneous field. Many others began experimenting with hysteroscopy in the '80s, leading to steady improvement of distending media and optical technology. But it was not until uterine septa were divided hysteroscopically that the explosion in transcervical hys-teroscopic approaches emerged. Today hysteroscopy is a valuable clinical tool. It allows for diagnosis and treatment of some of the most important and frequently encountered disease entities that the gynecologist manages, including dysfunctional uterine bleeding and postmenopausal bleeding.

Proper instrumentation is essential to good technique. Nowhere is this more obvious than in endoscopic procedures, where nothing replaces high-quality, technologically advanced instruments in accomplishing surgical goals. Today's instrumentation is highly sophisticated and requires constant maintenance; improvements based on innovative engineering breakthroughs occur continually. It is essential for the hysteroscopic surgeon to be adept with rigid hysteroscopes, flexible hysteroscopes, and the use of video.

I believe that the next wave of advancement in hysteroscopic surgery will be the introduction of these techniques to an office setting. Gynecologic surgeons have started to do endometrial ablation successfully in an office operatory, using mild sedation. As managed care becomes more influential and gynecologic practice is reoriented toward an ambulatory model, endoscopic procedures will become increasingly more prominent among techniques employed in the office operatory. It is difficult to tell which came first, i.e., did the ability to do endoscopic surgery facilitate the shift to office-based gynecologic practice or did the necessity to do office procedures instigate the growth in interest in endoscopic surgery, especially hysteroscopy?

Not as exciting as the advancements in hardware but noteworthy nonetheless are the changes in the use of distending media. Various distending media have been developed over time, starting with crystalloids, then Dextran 70, and now the use of glycine, sorbitol, and saline. CO_2 is used in the office because of its neatness, but all of these distending media are satisfactory. Surgeons must be able to move from one medium to another to accomplish their goals.

Among the achievements of this textbook are its successful combination of basic technique with a sophisticated and in-depth discussion of instrumentation and the inclusion of detailed instructions describing how to perform a variety of procedures, including diagnostic laparoscopy, endometrial ablation, removal of a uterine septum, and tubal canalization.

In addition to providing basic information and a "how-to" approach, the utility of any textbook is predicated on the recognition and discussion of complications. The contributors to this textbook have provided excellent examples and illustrations of complications together with discussions on how to avoid these pitfalls.

Office hysteroscopy is a procedure whose time has come. For many years, its utility was limited to diagnosis. But with the development of therapeutic hysteroscopic procedures that can be performed in the office setting at reduced cost, an avalanche of new techniques is sure to follow. We can look forward to many more breakthroughs that will make this type of surgery even more effective. I am most assured that in the area of ablation alone, we have just begun to scratch the surface.

Alan H. DeCherney, M.D.

PREFACE

Before the introduction of continuous-flow hysteroscopy in the 1980s, only a small percentage of practicing gynecologists truly visualized the uterine cavity. Because of this, many of the accepted therapies for intrauterine pathology were based on blind, random sampling of the endometrium. For example, when a woman suffered from menorrhagia to the point of anemia and the blind endometrial sampling showed benign tissue, then the only option for this patient was hysterectomy. It was only when the uterus was opened on the pathology table that it was discovered that many patients had suffered from one of a variety of intrauterine pathologies such as submucous myomata.

As physicians became experienced with panoramic hysteroscopy in the operating room, they began to perform more and more diagnostic and therapeutic procedures that are precisely directed at the pathology and are often uterine sparing. However, even today, less than half of the gynecologists in the United States are routinely performing diagnostic and/or therapeutic hysteroscopy. These percentages will most certainly change as physicians become more educated and experienced with hysteroscopy.

Although 20% of U.S. gynecologists perform hysteroscopy in the operating room, it is estimated that only 8% of U.S. gynecologists routinely perform office hysteroscopy. There are many reasons for this, but the most important factor is physician education. The primary goal of this book is to help physicians understand that office hysteroscopy is a cost-effective method of instant diagnosis that can change practice habits. As a practical guide to office hysteroscopy, this book will help physicians understand the indications for office hysteroscopy, decide on appropriate equipment needs, and provide a step-by-step guide through the procedure.

Much of this book is directed to physicians who want to perform diagnostic office hysteroscopy. Office hysteroscopy is far more specific than radiologic modalities, such as ultrasound, sonohysterography, magnetic resonance imaging, and hysterosalpingography, which require image interpretation. Many physicians have shied away from office hysteroscopy because of the misconception that it is a morbid procedure with a poor-quality image. With the small-diameter flexible hysteroscopes currently available, the endometrial cavity can be thoroughly evaluated in less than one minute without the need for a cervical tenaculum or local anesthesia. Many examples of the quality of image obtained with this technology are contained throughout the text.

For the advanced hysteroscopist and for surgeons who would like to perform more office-based therapeutic procedures, Drs. Gimpelson, Surrey, and Awwad have described a myriad of intrauterine procedures they are currently performing in the office. By no means have they described a complete list of these procedures. As technology advances the list of therapeutic office hysteroscopic procedures will grow. It is likely that the cost benefits of these procedures will become so overwhelming that insurance companies will soon demand that these techniques be performed in the office.

It is my firm belief that the office hysteroscope will be used in gynecology as commonly as the urologist uses a cystoscope and the otolaryngologist uses a naso-pharyngoscope. More than 700,000 blind diagnostic D&Cs were performed in the United States in 1993. With the use of the office hysteroscope, which can provide the surgeon with a specific diagnosis in a rapid, nonmorbid, and cost-effective fashion, blind procedures will be reduced to a fraction of their current number.

Keith B. Isaacson, M.D.

ACKNOWLEDGMENTS

I want to thank the Olympus Corporation for providing much of the hysteroscopic equipment needed to produce this text. I also thank Mr. Craig Traub for effectively communicating his strong beliefs in office hysteroscopy. Many thanks also go out to Ellen Baker Geisel (alias Marge S.) and Jane Stiller for their excellent administrative and editing skills.

CONTENTS

OFFICE HYSTEROSCOPY

Chapter 1

A HISTORY OF HYSTEROSCOPY

Maryse D. Roudier
Alan H. DeCherney

The first working endoscope was developed by Desormeaux[1] in 1865. This instrument was the first to allow visual inspection of internal organs. In 1869 Pantaleoni[2] used a device similar to Desormeaux's endoscope to view the interior of the uterus of a 60-year-old woman with therapy-resistant bleeding. With this endoscope, he was able to observe a polypoid growth and cauterize it with silver nitrate.

EARLY HYSTEROSCOPIC TECHNIQUES

Bumm[3] was one of the first physicians to extensively study hysteroscopy and its use in gynecology. At the Vienna Congress in 1895, he presented the results of a series of intrauterine endoscopic examinations that had been done with a modified urethroscope. With this instrument he had been able to diagnose conditions such as endometritis, carcinomas, or other lesions in the corpus despite bleeding that obscured the view. A headlamp with an incandescent light reflector served as an illuminator.

The era of modern hysteroscopy began with David's 1908 report.[4] David performed hysteroscopy using a cystoscope with an internal light and lens system. He was the first physician to fully describe the technique, indications, contraindications, dangers, and uses of the hysteroscope. David presented 25 uncomplicated cases in his report. His instrument consisted of a sheath into which was fitted a cystoscope closed at the far end by a glass crystal and with an incandescent lamp contained near it. A magnifying lens was attached to the ocular or near end. By enclosing the lamp, he was able to keep the visual field free of blood; by varying the size of the sheath according to the anatomy of the patient, he could minimize the need for anesthesia.

In 1914 Heineberg[5] published an account of his hysteroscopic method. His hysteroscope consisted of an internally illuminated endoscopic tube with a water-irrigating system surrounding the inner opening. The water was used to wash away obscuring blood. Heineberg performed 20 examinations, most with satisfactory results.

Rubin[6] published a paper in 1925 comparing the use of hysteroscopy with that of cystoscopy. Although the procedures resembled each other, hysteroscopy was still not as commonly used and accepted as cystoscopy. According to Rubin, the smallness of the uterine cavity itself and the problem of endometrial bleeding accounted for this discrepancy. To compensate for these two obstacles, Rubin suggested expanding the uterine cavity with carbon dioxide gas or dry air using a rubber bulb or syringe. In addition, he used the cystourethroscope (devised by McCarthy), which consisted of an outer sheath with the obturator in place and a well-rounded tip that facilitated insertion, causing less trauma to the endometrium and therefore less bleeding.[6]

Rubin discussed using a wider sheath that allowed the use of operating instruments such as scissors or fulguration wire. He also reported a method of amputating growths, for example, by sucking or pressing them into an oval window and rotating an outer sheath over this window to sever the base of the growth. In addition, Rubin[6] delineated the advantages and contraindications of hysteroscopy.

Rubin experimented with water irrigation and found that positive pressure was required to dislodge clots or clean the instrument tip. However, negative pressure was preferred because it was gentler. But after finding that negative pressure irrigation could neither remove coagulated blood nor had a hemostatic effect, Rubin abandoned water use altogether.[6]

In 1925 Seymour[7] reported using suction for removing blood during hysteroscopy. His hysteroscope resembled a bronchoscope. One channel contained a replaceable tubular light. Continuous suction was maintained through two other channels. Because the field of vision was limited, the examination had to be done in stages.

Von Mikulicz-Radecki and Freund[8] presented an account of their experiences with hysteroscopy in 1927. They used a water-rinsing system to keep the objective lens clean. Saline was pumped in through a tube. Because the saline mixed with blood (preventing adequate visualization), liquid was not used to dilate the uterine cavity. Von Mikulicz-Radecki and Freund[8] attempted catheterization of the fallopian tubes and obtained samples for biopsy under direct visualization with their hysteroscopic technique.

In 1928 Gauss[9] achieved adequate intrauterine visualization by means of an optical instrument into which a flow of liquid was directed from a height of 50 cm. The outflowing liquid was drained into a receptacle. Based on his experiences, Gauss was convinced that hysteroscopy would find wide application.

Schroeder,[10] a student of Gauss', continued his work and improved on the right-angle lens by making the optic system forward-viewing. He attempted one of the first hysteroscopic sterilizations using electrocoagulation. His first two cases both failed.

Norment et al[11] continued attempts to improve visualization during hysteroscopy. In 1957 they published a summary of their experiences and detailed his hysteroscopic technique. The development of their instrument spanned 18 years. Initially, an inflatable rubber bag over the objective lens was used to keep the uterus dilated. The rubber bag was transparent and in some cases allowed examination of the uterine cavity. In others, however, the bag became wrinkled and rendered direct inspection impossible. A few years later, this bag was replaced by a piece of transparent plastic. Blood and secretions were removed using a water-rinsing system.

In 1962 Silander[12] reported using a water-filled balloon to distend the uterine cavity and prevent bleeding. This technique was critized, however, because the balloon compressed the endometrium, altering its appearance.

The development of glass fiber optics during the later 1950s and early 1960s helped to advance hysteroscopy in particular and the field of endoscopy in general. In 1963 Mohri et al[13] introduced a hysterofiberscope that was used to observe intrauterine phenomena late in pregnancy. Although the fiberoptic hysteroscope may be useful for specific procedures, the major contribution of fiberoptics technology to operative hysteroscopy to date has been in providing a convenient, flexible light source.

IMPROVED METHODS FOR UTERINE DISTENTION

During the 1970s, various methods were introduced to improve uterine distention. In 1970 Edstrom and Fernstrom[14] reported their use of 32% dextran 70 and found it superior to previously described methods. Because of its high viscosity, 32% dextran 70 was not miscible with blood.

Examinations could be performed with good visibility even in the presence of a modest amount of blood, making 32% dextran 70 a useful distending medium for both diagnostic and operative hysteroscopy. However, complications caused by 32% dextran 70 did occur, including allergic reactions and rare pulmonary edema.[15,16] Levine and Neuwirth[17] used 30% dextran successfully. Lindemann[18] used carbon dioxide gas and a hysteroscope adapter he developed that fitted over the cervix to prevent escape of the gas. Early use of insufflation equipment in the uterus with high flow rates designed for laparoscopy resulted in cardiac arrhythmias and arrest.[19] When the insufflators were specially designed for hysteroscopy, however, this method became safe. Unfortunately, a disadvantage of carbon dioxide as a distention medium in operative blood was its tendency to mix with the blood. This mixing caused air bubbles that obscured the field. Other distention media that were found to be safe included 5% dextrose and saline. Their low viscosity made them miscible with blood and therefore not good media for operative hysteroscopy, where bleeding may occur.

ADVANCES IN OPERATIVE HYSTEROSCOPY

Improvements in uterine distention methods allowed operative hysteroscopy to further develop. In 1974 Edstrom[20] was one of the first physicians to describe the removal of an intrauterine device using the hysteroscope and strong, firmly attached forceps. Siegler and Kemmann[21] in 1976 reported the hysteroscopic removal of misplaced or embedded intrauterine devices using a grasping forceps through the operating channel. Finally, in 1977 Valle et al[22] used hysteroscopy to locate and remove intrauterine devices with missing filaments.

Besides removing intrauterine devices, hysteroscopy became the method of choice in the diagnosis and treatment of intrauterine adhesions. Levine and Neuwirth[23] used hysteroscopy and laparoscopy to evaluate 10 patients with hysterographic diagnosis of Asherman's syndrome. In four of these patients, synechiae were dissected through the hysteroscope using miniature scissors or an electrocautery probe. This report focused attention on important advantages gained with the use of the hysteroscope in patients with Asherman's syndrome. Hysteroscopy was more accurate than blind curettage or dissection and safer than laparotomy. Using laparoscopy in addition to hysteroscopy helped prevent uterine perforation. In 1974 Edstrom[20] reported an alternative technique in which a series of nine patients had intrauterine synechiae either ruptured by the endoscope or excised at the base and top with the biopsy forceps. March et al[24] published a paper in which 66 patients underwent hysteroscopic lysis of adhesions using miniature scissors. Short-term results were excellent. Of those patients studied postlysis of adhesions, 94% had a normal uterine cavity. In 1978 Sugimoto[25] reported hysteroscopic adhesiolysis using the outer sleeve of the hysteroscope to break the adhesion under visual control. In both Sugimoto's and March's series,[25,26] the pregnancy rate among patients who wished to conceive was greater than the pregnancy rate achieved with earlier therapeutic modalities, such as repeat curettage or hysterotomy.

In addition to lysing intrauterine adhesions, hysteroscopy was used in the development of new myomectomy techniques. Norment et al[11] were among the first physicians to describe a loop for resecting wide-based polyps and submucosal fibroids. No specific cases were reported.

In 1976 Neuwirth and Amin[27] reported five cases of transcervical removal of submucosal fibroids in which hysteroscopic guidance was used. All of the cases involved pedunculated fibroids; the pedicles were cut with scissors or twisted off using ovum forceps. A "new" hysteroscopic technique for removal of sessile submucosal fibroids was described 2 years later.[28] Neuwirth used a modified urologic resectoscope that was adapted to the higher pressures necessary in 32% dextran 70 hysteroscopy. A cutting loop that moved to and fro beyond the telescope was used. Four patients were treated in this manner. DeCherney and Polan[29] (1983) removed both pedunculated and sessile myomas less than 3 cm in diameter using an unmodified urologic resectoscope. No immediate or later complications developed.

Hysteroscopic methods for female sterilization have also been developed but none has found widespread use. Between 1953 and 1969, Hayashi[30] designed electrodes capable of coagulating the fallopian tubes under the control of hysteroscopy or fluoroscopy. Results were poor, with pregnancy rates ranging from 5% to 83%. Quinones Guerror et al[31] and Richart et al[32] published reports on clinical trials using hysteroscopically directed electrodes to fulgurate the uterine tubal openings. Although initial results were encouraging, subsequent reports of high failure rates and significant complications led to the abandonment of this technique.[33,34,35]

In 1976 Lindemann and Mohr[36] used hysteroscopy to inject a chemical used for tubal occlusion, methyl-2-cyanoacrylate (MCA), into the oviducts of 150 women. Several other agents have been used in attempts to achieve permanent tubal occlusion, but none has found widespread clinical use.

Investigators have also attempted to provide reversible tubal occlusion via the hysteroscope. In 1979 Reed and Erb[37] described a procedure in which formed-in-place silicone rubber plugs were placed hysteroscopically. An update of their experience 2 years later showed an overall success rate for bilateral occlusion of 71.5% (239 women).[38] With improvements, the bilateral occlusion rate increased to 92.3% (25 patients). The authors found that proper case selection was important and estimated that approximately 10% of patients would not be considered good candidates for the procedure because of anatomic reasons.[38]

Excision of uterine septa was also reported to result in a high rate of reproductive success without the associated risks of more traditional therapies. Edstrom[20] described resection of uterine septa in two cases using a hysteroscopic

technique. Chervenak and Neuwrith[39] described a new approach, using hysteroscopic resection under laparoscopic control. Two cases were reported in which very fine scissors were used to resect the septa. Bleeding was controlled by focal cautery using a coagulating current. Daly et al[40] reported 14 patients with uterine septa who underwent hysteroscopic septal divisions. In these cases, small scissors were used to incise the septa. Laparoscopy was used to monitor the depth of resection. A year later, DeCherney and Polan[29] reported 11 patients with intrauterine septa less than 1 cm at the broadest point that were resected using an unmodified urologic cystoscope. Nine patients carried a fetus to term during the 5- to 25-month follow-up. March incised 91 septa using flexible scissors under hysteroscopic guidance. Most septa were 3 to 5 cm in depth and width. Two were 8 cm wide. A total of 79 patients had had a history of recurrent abortion. Their gestational outcome post-therapy markedly improved.[41]

The treatment of intractable uterine bleeding has also been approached recently by hysteroscopy. Goldrath et al[42] first reported on 22 patients who had excessive and disabling uterine bleeding and were treated with hysteroscopic endometrial ablation using neodymium:yttrium aluminum garnet (Nd:YAG) laser photovaporization. Successful results were obtained for 21 patients. The longest period of observation was 23 months. The one failure occurred in an anticoagulated patient with an artificial mitral valve. The Nd:YAG was chosen over other lasers because of its greater energy output, degree of tissue damage, and portability, facilitating its use in the operating room. DeCherney and Polan[29] used an unmodified urologic resectoscope to cauterize the entire endometrial surface in patients with intractable uterine bleeding unresponsive to hormonal therapy. Results up to 18 months later were good. In 1987 DeCherney et al[43] reported a series of 21 patients who had undergone hysteroscopic endometrial ablation using the resectoscope; 18 of the patients had blood dyscrasias or were poor anesthetic risks. The follow-up period ranged from 6 months to 5 years. The technique was noted to be efficient and beneficial.

The role of lasers in operative hysteroscopy continues to be explored. The argon and potassium titanyl phosphate 532 (KTP-532) lasers have less depth of penetration than the Nd:YAG laser, but their properties include a fiber delivery system and the ability to pass through fluid. Both lasers can be used in the uterus. Diamond et al[44] used the KTP-532 laser to lyse intrauterine adhesions and partially treat extensive intracavitary uterine fibroids. The laser was easy to use but required sophisticated equipment, including specialized electrical wiring, in the operating room. The relative usefulness of laser vs. nonlaser operative techniques remains to be established.

"I believe the real future of hysteroscopy is in office diagnosis and treatment of abnormal uterine bleeding," Corson[45] wrote in 1983. In 1981 Corson began using the Hamou microcolpohysteroscope and found that he was generally able to perform biopsies using an aspiration cannula or polyp forceps without anesthesia. Taylor and Hamou[46] went even further by stating that "all types of hysteroscopy [could] be performed in the office." In a series of 959 cases of microhysteroscopy, no anesthesia was used. The majority of the patients had less discomfort than that caused by hysterosalpingography, with a little less than half comparing the discomfort to that of menstruation.[47]

In 1985 Goldrath and Sherman[48] concluded that office hysteroscopy and suction curettage were more convenient, safer, and less expensive than the traditional diagnostic dilatation and curettage used to evaluate abnormal uterine conditions. In a series of 406 patients, there were no infections and no uterine perforations. Diagnostic accuracy seemed to be enhanced with the hysteroscopic method. Finally, hysteroscopy and suction curettage in an office setting saved more than $1000 per patient when compared with an outpatient hospital procedure. When compared with an inpatient hospital procedure, the savings were even greater.

In 1990 Lin et al[49] published their experience with a series of 1503 patients using the Fujinon diagnostic fiber optic hysteroscope. This endoscope, developed with the support of the Fuji Photo Optical Company in 1985, comprised three sections—a soft flexible anterior end, a rigid middle, and a soft posterior end. The scope had a diameter of 3.7 mm with a bending capacity of 100° up and 90° down. These characteristics allowed the scope to be used easily in an office setting without a tenaculum, cervical dilation, or anesthesia, even in nulliparous women. As a result, no complications were encountered during or after the procedure.

CONCLUSION

Over the past two decades, hysteroscopy has become widely implemented. It has been useful in the localization of intrauterine devices for later removal. The hysteroscope has been used in patients with infertility in conjunction with laparoscopy to further delineate the etiology of the infertility. Other uses include the treatment of uterine bleeding and Asherman's syndrome and as a means for sterilization. Hysteroscopy allows for the direct visualization of the endometrial cavity, thereby avoiding diagnostic errors associated with blind dilatation and curettage and endometrial biopsies. Use of the hysteroscope is growing rapidly and is a skill that gynecologists should have, especially because hysteroscopy is expected to become a common office procedure in the future. Performed as an outpatient procedure under local or no anesthesia, there is not only a decrease in morbidity but also a decrease in hospitalization and related costs. In this era of managed costs, such advantages are an important consideration.

REFERENCES

1. Desormeaux A-J: De l'endoscope et de ses applications au diagnostic et au traitement des affections de l'urethra et de la vessie, *Baillieres Clin Obstet Gynaecol* Paris, 1865.
2. Pantaleoni DC: On endoscopic examination of the cavity of the womb, *Med Press Circ* 8:26-27, 1869.
3. Bumm E: Zur aetiologie der endometritis, *Verhandlungen der Deutschen Gessellschaft fur Gynakologie* 6:524, 1895.
4. David C: L'endoscopie uterine (hysteroscopie): applications au diagnostic et au traitement des affections intrauterines. In Jaques G, Ed: *These de Paris,* Paris, 1908.
5. Heineberg A: Uterine endoscopy: an aid to precision in the diagnosis of intrauterine disease, a preliminary report, with the presentation of a new uteroscope, *Surgery, Gynecology and Obstetrics* 18:513-515, 1914.
6. Rubin IC: Uterine endoscopy, endometroscopy with the aid of uterine insufflation, *Am J Obstet Gynecol* 10(3):313-327, 1925.
7. Seymour HJ: Endoscopy of the uterus: with a description of hysteroscopy, *British Medical Journal* 2:1220, 1925.
8. Von Mikulicz-Radecki F, Freund A: Ein neues Hysteroskop und sein praktische Anwendung in der Gynakologie, *Zeitschrift fur Geburtshilfe und Gynakologie,* 1927.
9. Gauss CJ: Hysteroskopie, *Archiv fur Gynakologie* 133:18, 1928.
10. Schroeder C: Uber den Ausbau und die Leistungen der Hysteroskopie, *Archiv fur Gynakologie* 156:407, 1934.
11. Norment WB et al: Hysteroscopy, *Surg Clin North Am* 37:1377-1386, 1957.
12. Silander T: Hysteroscopy through a transparent rubber balloon, *Surgery, Gynecology and Obstetrics* 114:125-127, 1962.
13. Mohri T, Mohri C, Yamadori F: The original production of the glass-fibre hysteroscope and a study on the intrauterine observation of the human fetus, things attached to the fetus and inner side of the uterus wall in late pregnancy and the beginning of delivery by means of hysteroscopy and its recording on the film, *Journal of the Japanese Obstetrics and Gynecology Society* 15(2):87-95, 1986.
14. Edstrom K, Fernstrom I: The diagnostic possibilities of a modified hysteroscopic technique, *Acta Obstet Gynecol Scand* 49:327-330, 1970.
15. Maddi VI, Wyso EM, Zinner EN: Dextran anaphylaxis, *Angiology* 20:243, 1969.
16. Leake JL, Murphy AA, Zacur EN: Noncardiogenic pulmonary edema: a complication of operative hysteroscopy, *Fertil Steril* 48:497-499, 1987.
17. Levine RU, Neuwirth RS: Evaluation of a method of hysteroscopy with the use of 30% dextran, *Am J Obstet Gynecol* 113:696, 1972.
18. Lindemann HJ: Historical aspects of hysteroscopy, *Fertil Steril* 24(3):230-243, 1973.
19. Porto R: Hysteroscopie, *Encyclopedie medico-chirurgicale* Paris, 1974, Searle Laboratories/Clin-Comar-Byla.
20. Edstrom KGB: Intrauterine surgical procedures during hysteroscopy, *Endoscopy* 6:175-181, 1974.
21. Siegler AM, Kemmann E: Location and removal of misplaced or embedded intrauterine devices by hysteroscopy, *J Reprod Med* 16(3):139-144, 1976.
22. Valle RF, Sciarra FF, Freeman DW: Hysteroscopic removal of intrauterine devices with missing filaments, *Obstet Gynecol* 49(1):55-60, 1977.
23. Levine RU, Neuwirth RS: Simultaneous laparoscopy and hysteroscopy for intrauterine adhesions, *Obstet Gynecol* 42(3):441-445, 1973.
24. March CM, Israel R, March AD: Hysteroscopic management of intrauterine adhesions, *Am J Obstet Gynecol* 130(6):653-657, 1978.
25. Sugimoto O: Diagnostic and therapeutic hysteroscopy for traumatic intrauterine adhesions, *Am J Obstet Gynecol* 131(5):539-547, 1978.
26. March CM, Israel R: Gestational outcome following hysteroscopic lysis of adhesions, *Fertil Steril* 36(4):455-459, 1981.
27. Neuwirth RS, Amin HK: Excision of submucous fibroids with hysteroscopic control, *Am J Obstet Gynecol* 126(1):95-99, 1976.
28. Neuwirth RS: A new technique for and additional experience with hysteroscopic resection of submucous fibroids, *Am J Obstet Gynecol* 131(1):91-94, 1978.
29. DeCherney A, Polan ML: Hysteroscopic management of intrauterine lesions and intractable uterine bleeding, *Obstet Gynecol* 61(3):392-397, 1983.

30. Hayashi M: Tubal sterilization by cornual coagulation under hysteroscopy. In Richart RM, Praeger DJ, Eds: *Human sterilization* Springfield, Mass, 1972, Charles C Thomas.

31. Quinones Guerror R, Ramos RA, Duran AA: Tubal electrocauterization under hysteroscopic control, *Contraception* 7:195-201, 1973.

32. Richart RM et al: Female sterilization by electrocoagulation of tubal ostia using hysteroscopy, *Am J Obstet Gynecol* 117:801-804, 1973.

33. Richart RM: Complications of hysteroscopic sterilization, *Contraception* 10:230, 1974.

34. Cibils LA: Permanent sterilization by hysteroscopic cauterization, *Am J Obstet Gynecol* 121:513-520, 1975.

35. March CM, Israel R: A critical appraisal of hysteroscopic tubal fulguration for sterilization, *Contraception* 11:261-269, 1975.

36. Lindemann HJ, Mohr J: Review of clinical experience with hysteroscopic sterilization, In Sciarra JJ, Droegemueller W, Speidel JJ, Eds: *Advances in female sterilization techniques,* Hagerstown, 1976, Harper and Row.

37. Reed TP, Erb RA: Hysteroscopic oviductal blocking with formed-in-place silicone rubber plugs, *J Reprod Med* 23(2):69-72, 1979.

38. Reed TP, Erb RA, DeMaeyer J: Tubal occlusion with silicone rubber, Update, 1980. *J Reprod Med* 26(10):534-537, 1981.

39. Chervenak FA, Neuwirth RS: Hysteroscopic resection of the uterine septum, *Am J Obstet Gynecol* 141(3):351-353, 1981.

40. Daly DC et al: Hysteroscopic resection of uterine septa, *Surg Forum* 33:637-639, 1982.

41. March CM, Israel R: Hysteroscopic management of recurrent abortion caused by septate uterus, *Am J Obstet Gynecol* 156:834-842, 1987.

42. Goldrath MH, Fuller TA, Segal S: Laser photovaporization of endometrium for the treatment of menorrhagia, *Am J Obstet Gynecol* 140(1):14-19, 1981.

43. DeCherney AH et al: Endometrial ablation for intractable uterine bleeding: hysteroscopic resection, *Obstet Gynecol* 70:668-670, 1987.

44. Diamond MP et al: Endoscopic use of the potassium-titanyl-phosphate 532 laser in gynecologic surgery, Colposcopy and Gynecologic Laser Surgery 3(4):213-216, 1987.

45. Corson SL: Editorial comments: Clinical perspectives: hysteroscopy, *J Reprod Med* 28:388-389, 1983.

46. Taylor PJ, Hamou JE: Clinical perspectives: hysteroscopy, *J Reprod Med* 28:359-388, 1983.

47. Hamou J, Taylor PJ: Hysteroscopy, contact hysteroscopy and micro-colpohysteroscopy in gynecologic practice, *Curr Prob Obstet Gynecol* 6:17, 1982.

48. Goldrath MH, Sherman AI: Office hysteroscopy and suction curettage: Can we eliminate the hospital diagnostic dilatation and curettage? *Am J Obstet Gynecol* 152:220-229, 1985.

49. Lin B-L et al: The Fujinon Diagnostic Fiber Optic Hysteroscope: Experience with 1,503 patients, *J Reprod Med* 35: 685-689, 1990.

Chapter 2

INDICATIONS AND CONTRAINDICATIONS FOR OFFICE HYSTEROSCOPY

Louise Lapensee
Jay M. Cooper
Patricia A. Caplinger

Hysteroscopy is indicated in any situation in which intrauterine visualization will enhance diagnostic accuracy and refine therapy. The primary indication for diagnostic hysteroscopy, the evaluation of patients with abnormal bleeding, has not changed in the 126 years since Pantaleoni[1] performed the first hysteroscopic examination in 1869. In an attempt to find the cause for abnormal bleeding in a postmenopausal patient, Pantaleoni used a hollow tube (12.0 mm in diameter), reflective candlelight, and concave mirrors to examine the intrauterine cavity. Remarkably, despite this primitive instrumentation, he observed a blackberry-sized lesion, which may have been a polyp or carcinoma.

Present-day hysteroscopic instrumentation allows for excellent illumination, distention, and visualization of the endometrial cavity, obviating many of the problems Pantaleoni and physicians of earlier times experienced. A wide array of telescopes, both rigid and flexible, in addition to therapeutic hysteroscopic instrumentation, have made hysteroscopy an integral part of the gynecologist's armamentarium. Because many gynecologic conditions are now amenable to operative hysteroscopic techniques, it is imperative that gynecologists make the correct diagnoses by offering their patients diagnostic hysteroscopy.

To understand the hysteroscopic findings of pathologic lesions, physicians must first be able to recognize the variations of normal findings in uteri during both proliferative and secretory phases of the menstrual cycle and in the postmenopausal state. During the proliferative phase, the endometrium appears yellow-red with little or no evidence of surface blood vessels. The endometrium is thin but has some gentle undulation. Each tubal ostium is clearly seen at the apex of the cornu. The thin endometrium is somewhat resistant to bleeding but may do so if sufficiently traumatized. The endometrium during the secretory phase is thick, easily indentable, and traumatized. Occasional polypoid projections of engorged endometrium project into the cavity. Coiled vessels are often visible through the thick stroma. The endometrium of a normal postmenopausal uterus is thin and atrophied. The glandular openings are absent, the yellow-tan endometrium is uniformly flat, and small fragile blood vessels are easily seen.[2]

True pathology is rarely found in uteri of women who are asymptomatic for either abnormal bleeding or infertility.[3] The incidence of pathology found at hysteroscopic examination in a symptomatic patient population will vary depending on several factors, including patient age and the aggressiveness of the physician in initiating hysteroscopic examination early in the diagnostic evaluation.[4,5]

The best view of the uterine cavity is obtained with the distal lens in the lower uterine segment. The endometrium, the cavity's general structure, and the presence of any abnormalities such as polyps, myomas, or synechiae will be readily observed. Advancement and rotation of the hysteroscope allows for adequate visualization of both right and left uterine cornua and tubal ostia. Closer and magnified inspection of suspected pathology (i.e., adenomyosis, hyperplasia, endometritis, polyps, myomas, cancer, adhesions, or septa) is achieved by moving the scope closer to the abnormalities. Touching the distal lens to the lesion, and then withdrawing, will often allow the examiner to make a differential diagnosis between a polyp and a myoma. The endocervical canal is often better visualized while the telescope is being removed at the end of the examination rather than when it is first inserted.

As the physician gains more experience, the in-office diagnostic evaluation can be extended to allow for operative or therapeutic techniques as discussed in detail in Chapter 10. With appropriate equipment, pedunculated polyps generally can be removed in the office setting unless the entire uterine cavity is occupied by the polyp. Small pedunculated myomas can easily be removed in the office. Retained products of conception often cause persistent bleeding, and this problem can also be treated in an office setting.[4,6,7] Most operative procedures (i.e., submucous myomectomy, extensive polypectomy, and endometrial ablation) should be reserved

for an outpatient surgical facility where general anesthesia, larger diameter instruments, and continuous flow of low-viscosity fluid for uterine distention is available.

As gynecologists gain experience with diagnostic hysteroscopy, they will find a remarkably high degree of correlation between their clinical impression and the pathologist's histologic diagnosis of biopsy tissue. Consequently, the physician may be tempted, in cases where the cavity appears normal, to forego tissue sampling. This temptation should be avoided given the current liability climate in medical practice.

OVERVIEW OF INDICATIONS FOR OFFICE HYSTEROSCOPY

A partial list of indications for office hysteroscopy can be found in the box below. A complete list is not practical because the number of conditions for which office hysteroscopy can be applied is growing constantly. The most common indication for office hysteroscopy remains the evaluation of patients with abnormal uterine bleeding. Appropriate cases include abnormal uterine bleeding in pre-

---

Indications for office hysteroscopy

Evaluation of abnormal uterine bleeding

Premenopausal ovulatory women
Premenopausal anovulatory women who fail hormonal
    therapy
Postmenopausal women
FINDINGS
Submucous/intramural myomata
Endometrial polyps
Endometrial hyperplasia
Endometrial cancer
Adenomyosis
IUD

Infertility evaluation

Routine infertility
Abnormal hysterosalpingogram
Pre-IVF evaluation
Recurrent spontaneous abortions
FINDINGS
Submucous/intramural myomata
Endometrial polyps
Asherman's syndrome
Proximal tubal obstruction
Intratubal adhesions (falloposcopy)
Tubal cannulation for GIFT
Congenital uterine anormalies
    Septate or bicornuate uterus
    Uterus didelphys or unicollis

Localization of IUDs and foreign bodies

Evaluation of the pregnant patient

FINDINGS
IUD in pregnancy
Embryoscopy
Localization of placental implantation site
    Ectopic pregnancy (tubal or interstitial)
    Failed termination of pregnancy
    Difficult D&C
    Postpartum hemorrhage

Cervical examination (Hamou microcolpohysteroscope)

FINDINGS
Endocervical polyps
Visualization of squamocolumnar junction in unsatisfactory
    colposcopy
Vascular changes (in squamoepithelial lesions [SIL])

Postoperative evaluation

Hysteroscopic myomectomy
Abdominal myomectomy
Cesarean section
Septum repair
Asherman's repair
FINDINGS
De novo or recurrent intrauterine adhesions
Incomplete myoma resection

Endometrial carcinoma

FINDINGS
Staging
Second look after nonsurgical treatment

Tubal occlusion to effect sterilization

menopausal ovulatory women, failed hormonal treatment in premenopausal anovulatory women, and any abnormal uterine bleeding in postmenopausal women. Other indications for office hysteroscopy in women with abnormal uterine bleeding include menorrhagia induced by intrauterine devices (IUDs) and abnormal uterine bleeding in women with known cervical polyps.

Office hysteroscopy can be very useful in an infertility practice. It can be used to evaluate women with suspected Asherman's syndrome, women with suspected congenital uterine anomalies, and women with histories of recurrent first-trimester abortions or second- or early third-trimester pregnancy losses. Office hysteroscopy is also indicated in the workup of a patient about to enter an assisted reproductive technology (ART) program such as in vitro fertilization (IVF). Other indications related to infertility diagnosis and treatment include the evaluation and treatment of suspected proximal tubal occlusion, the evaluation of the tubal lumen using falloposcopy, and the treatment of infertility by hysteroscopic gamete intrafallopian transfer (GIFT), zygote intrafallopian transfer (ZIFT), or tubal embryo transfer (TET).

Additional but less frequent indications for office hysteroscopy include locating nonvisualized IUD strings and suspected intrauterine foreign bodies. During pregnancy, office hysteroscopy is used for the removal of an IUD in early pregnancy, for performing embryoscopy, for locating a pregnancy in failed terminations or difficult D&Cs, for postpartum hemorrhage, and for the diagnosis and treatment of tubal ectopic pregnancies especially in cases of suspected interstitial pregnancy.

Office hysteroscopy is useful in assessing uterine defects in patients with prior uterine surgical procedures such as cesarean sections, hysterotomies, or myomectomies, as well as the evaluation of the endocervical canal. Office hysteroscopy is being used more frequently for the evaluation of patients with suspected endometrial carcinoma. Several investigators have attempted and are currently investigating office hysteroscopy as a tool to perform tubal occlusion by chemical or mechanical methods to effect sterilization.

All of these indications will be discussed in more detail below. The purpose of this chapter is not only to list the indications for office hysteroscopy but also to inform the reader about the type of lesions that can be expected for a particular indication.

ABNORMAL UTERINE BLEEDING

Historically, gynecologists have offered their patients a D&C as a means to both diagnose and treat symptoms of abnormal uterine bleeding. It is remarkable how many women in their fifth or sixth decade of life report having undergone at least one D&C. For many patients, no diagnostic or therapeutic benefit is realized from a D&C. Because of physician and patient frustration, as well as the absence of long-term benefits, a hysterectomy often follows a failed D&C. That a blindly directed curettage of the endometrial cavity

rarely offers long-term therapeutic benefit is not a new concept.[5,8,9] There are few gynecologists who have not received from the pathologist, a diagnosis of endometrial polyps or submucous myomas after performing a hysterectomy in a patient who had had one or more "negative" D&Cs. Many authors have noted that a D&C is a poor method for evaluating the endometrial cavity.[5,6,9] Although a D&C is satisfactory for sampling endometrium to determine the hormonal status of the patient (i.e., proliferative or secretory phase), it will on occasion miss focal areas of hyperplasia or carcinoma.[2,5,8,9] Furthermore, endometrial polyps are often missed entirely or only partially sampled, and submucous myomas are virtually undiagnosable by D&C. In contrast, panoramic diagnostic hysteroscopy minimizes the relatively high error rate associated with a blind D&C. Additionally, hysteroscopy has been shown to be superior to hysterosalpingography in the evaluation of the patient experiencing irregular vaginal bleeding, reducing an estimated false positive error rate of 30%.[8,10]

Office hysteroscopy should be strongly considered in all ovulatory women with abnormal uterine bleeding, in those who are anovulatory and have had a failed course of medical treatment, or when an underlying anatomic cause is suspected.[11] Office hysteroscopy should also be performed to evaluate women who have postmenopausal bleeding with or without the use of hormone replacement therapy.

Between 40% and 85% of patients with abnormal bleeding will demonstrate a uterine abnormality at hysteroscopy. Myomas and polyps can be a cause of dysmenorrhea, abnormal bleeding, and infertility. The false diagnostic rate associated with hysterosalpingography provides a valid reason to perform hysteroscopy because even a D&C may not recognize or adequately treat either of these two abnormalities. Ultrasonography may accurately map the extent of the myoma, but often cannot distinguish between a myoma and a polyp.[12] Vercellini et al[13] performed hysteroscopy in 61 consecutive premenopausal women with abnormal uterine bleeding and moderate to severe iron-deficiency anemia. Benign disease was found in 41 (67%) subjects including submucous myomas, intramural/subserous myomas, endometrial polyps, and adenomyosis. In the other 20 (33%), no organic lesions were found. Fifteen of these 20 women were anovulatory, and their abnormal bleeding was therefore hormonally related. Transvaginal sonography failed to detect 15% of intrauterine lesions. Fedele et al[14] performed hysteroscopy and transvaginal ultrasound in 71 women hospitalized for hysterectomy. They all had symptomatic uterine myomas diagnosed by pelvic examination and abdominal ultrasound. Of the 71 patients, 18% were found to have submucous myomas. Hysteroscopy had a sensitivity and a specificity of 100% and 96% respectively. An abnormal hysteroscopic test had a predictive value of 87% whereas that of a normal test was 100%. Hysteroscopy was superior to transvaginal sonography in differentiating submucous myomas and endometrial polyps. Based on these results, it would seem that the main use of transvaginal sonography should be for screening whereas hysteroscopy should constitute the definitive diagnostic test. Cicinelli et al[15] compared transvaginal sonography, transabdominal sonohysterography, and hysteroscopy for the diagnosis and evaluation of submucous myomas in 52 premenopausal women hospitalized for hysterectomy. Both sonohysterography and hysteroscopy had a sensitivity, specificity, and predictive value of 100% for the diagnosis of submucous myomas.

Office hysteroscopy is a valuable tool in evaluating women with IUD-induced menorrhagia. Lei and Xie[16] performed hysteroscopy, hysterosalpingography, and ultrasonography in 105 of these women and found that endometrium and/or the location of the IUD were abnormal in 46 cases (43.8%). When a normal endometrium was noted, there was a 100% correlation in the findings by all three modalities. However, when abnormalities were noted, the correlation of hysterography and ultrasonography with hysteroscopy was only 25%. Hysteroscopy should then be considered in all cases of IUD-induced menorrhagia, especially if no abnormal findings are observed using ultrasound or hysterography.

Cervical polyps are often incidental findings at routine gynecologic examinations but can cause abnormal bleeding and have been associated with endometrial lesions, mainly endometrial polyps. Coeman et al[17] performed hysteroscopy in 165 patients with a cervical polyp. Forty-two (25.4%) cervical polyps were associated with a history of abnormal vaginal bleeding; the others were incidental findings. Endometrial polyps were found in 26.7% of patients, with a lower incidence (8.3%) in women undergoing a combined oral contraceptive pill treatment. Postmenopausal patients had a 56.8% incidence of cervix-related endometrial polyps. Hormone replacement therapy or abnormal vaginal bleeding did not significantly increase the incidence of coexisting polyps. Iossa et al,[18] in a retrospective study of 2007 consecutive office hysteroscopies, performed 442 procedures for the presence of cervical polyps. They found no cases of endometrial cancer. Office hysteroscopy should therefore be considered in the evaluation of any woman with a cervical polyp and associated abnormal vaginal bleeding or in postmenopausal women with cervical polyps.

D&C remains today the most commom diagnostic modality in the evaluation of postmenopausal bleeding despite reports concerning its hazards and its widely reported lack of diagnostic precision for malignant conditions.[19] The cost savings of hysteroscopy compared with a D&C have been reported. An estimated $1000 is saved per office-setting hysteroscopy and biopsy compared with a hospital procedure that uses an operating room and ancillary staff for pre and postoperative observation.[12] Altaras et al[19] studied 39 postmenopausal women in whom D&C had failed to obtain an adequate endometrial sample and performed hysteroscopy followed by an endometrial biopsy. Histopathology results were available for diagnosis in

74.3% (29/39) of the cases. Among these, 62% (18/29) had abnormal pathologic findings, including three cases (16.6% [3/18]) of endometrial carcinoma. Submucous fibroids were noted in 10 patients (25.6% [10/39]). The sensitivity, specificity, and predictive value for hysteroscopy alone were found to be 93.7%, 76%, and 83.3% respectively. Cacciatore et al[20] compared prospectively transvaginal sonography and hysteroscopy with D&C findings in 45 women who had postmenopausal bleeding with or without use of hormone replacement therapy. Hysteroscopy was successfully performed in 95.6% of cases. Using histologic findings from the D&C as the gold standard, authors found that the hysteroscopy had a sensitivity of 86.9%, a specificity of 91.7%, and a positive predictive value of 90.9%. Townsend et al[21] evaluated 110 women with persistent postmenopausal bleeding with or without hormone replacement therapy. A total of 95 women were found to have a benign organic lesion (polyps in 42 cases and submucous myoma in 53 cases), 13 had no disease, and 2 had early adenocarcinoma. In those patients without an organic cause, adenomyosis was found on uterine biopsy in eight and atrophic changes were noted in five. Downes and Al-Azzawi[22] performed outpatient hysteroscopy in 254 postmenopausal women with abnormal bleeding while taking hormone replacement therapy. They found a high incidence (47.6%) of structural lesions.

In women experiencing difficulties with hormone replacement therapy, hysteroscopy can improve long-term compliance by detecting lesions that may be amenable to treatment. This finding emphasizes the importance of office hysteroscopy as part of the evaluation of women with postmenopausal bleeding.

When diagnostic in-office hysteroscopy is performed early in the evaluation of a patient with abnormal uterine bleeding, anxiety is quickly allayed, a correct diagnosis is promptly made, and unnecessary laboratory tests and hormonal therapy are avoided.

LOCALIZATION OF IUDS AND FOREIGN BODIES

Office diagnostic hysteroscopy is particularly valuable for evaluating the patient wearing an IUD in which the string is not seen or felt at the cervical os.[23] Generally, this finding is indicative not of an unrecognized expulsion or penetration of the device into the peritoneal cavity, but rather of the string having been pulled up into the uterine cavity. During diagnostic hysteroscopy, under direct vision, the string of the device can be grasped and brought through the cervix into the vagina. Employing this approach, unnecessary flat plate radiologic examination and blind, painful probing of the uterine cavity can be avoided. If part of the IUD is broken during retrieval, hysteroscopy will usually be required to identify the position of the missing piece.[12] Hysteroscopy is also useful in diagnosing and treating intrauterine foreign bodies. Marcus et al[24] reported two cases of endometrial ossification presenting as secondary infertility in which diagnosis and removal were performed by hysteroscopy. Borgatta and Barrad[25] reported a case in which hysteroscopy and recovery of fragments of *Laminaria* were performed after an intrauterine *Laminaria* was crushed and removed 15 months earlier. The authors recommended a follow-up hysteroscopy be considered after fragmentation of all retained *Laminaria*.

EVALUATION

The infertile patient

The hysteroscope is ideal for in-office diagnostic evaluation of the infertile patient, the patient with suspected Asherman's syndrome, and the patient with a history of habitual spontaneous abortion. Intrauterine pathology has been reported in 10% to 62% of infertile couples.[26] In patients suspected of having space-occupying lesions of the endometrial cavity, diagnostic hysteroscopy has been shown to be superior to both hysterosalpingography and curettage.[4,5,9,27,28] Golan et al[29] found that hysterosalpingography had a specificity of 23%, a false positive rate of 44%, and a false negative rate of 10% compared with hysteroscopy in 152 women referred for IVF with a suspicion of an intrauterine abnormality on a previous hysterosalpingogram. Hysteroscopy has been recommended in the investigation of all patients with infertility and should be part of the workup in all patients undergoing IVF.[12]

Although the diagnosis of intrauterine synechiae, described by Asherman, is often suggested by a hysterosapingogram, as well as the patient's reproductive history (i.e., the onset of amenorrhea or hypomenorrhea and/or secondary infertility following a curettage during or after pregnancy), only hysteroscopy can enable one to make a definitive diagnosis. Diagnostic hysteroscopy allows the gynecologist to grade the severity of the adhesions and therefore map out a therapeutic plan that will likely return the patient to a fertile state. The most widely employed classification system of intrauterine adhesions is that of March, Israel, and March.[30] Minimal adhesions are defined as those that occupy less than one fourth of the uterine cavity. The adhesions are thin or filmy, and the ostial areas and the upper fundus are either minimally involved or clear of adhesions. A moderately severe case is one in which a fourth to three fourths of the uterine cavity is involved. There is no evidence of agglutination of the endometrial walls (only adhesions are present) and the ostial areas and upper fundus are only partially occluded. In severe cases of intrauterine adhesions, more than three fourths of the uterine cavity is involved, agglutination of the walls or thick bands are noted, and the ostial areas and upper cavity are virtually occluded. Thin, filmy adhesions can often be lysed at the time of the diagnostic examination; however, thicker, more tenacious and laterally placed adhesive bands require a meticulous operative hysteroscopic procedure under general anesthesia and often require laparoscopic control to avoid inadvertent uterine perforation.

Diagnostic hysteroscopy is an invaluable tool for patients suspected of having a septate or two-chambered uterus.[2,8,10] When combined with laparoscopy, hysteroscopy can differentiate the septate from the bicornuate uterus. A uterine septum has no typical appearance. It may extend as far down as the cervix, in which case the hysteroscope can be inserted into one side only. Given that, one must be careful not to make a false diagnosis of unicollis uterus. The absence of an intrauterine septum and the presence of a normal cavity can be made only after both tubal ostia or cornual tubal recesses are visualized. When only one os is seen in a rather cylindrically shaped fundus, an entry into the other side must be diligently pursued. In cases where diagnostic hysteroscopy confirms evidence of a septate uterus, operative hysteroscopic resection of the septum can be considered.[31] Should this procedure be undertaken, a concomitant diagnostic laparoscopic examination must be performed to rule out the possibility of a uterus didelphys, as well as help reduce the risk of uterine perforation.

Diagnostic hysteroscopy should be performed in the evaluation of patients with recurrent pregnancy loss of the first trimester or after one second-trimester or early third-trimester loss. Up to 33% of infertile couples with recurrent pregnancy loss are found to have intrauterine pathology.[26] Raziel et al[32] prospectively performed hysterosalpingography and office hysteroscopy in 106 patients with a history of at least three recurrent abortions. The hystero-salpingogram showed some abnormality of the uterine cavity in 60 patients (56.6%); 50 patients (47%) had an abnormal hysteroscopy. Compared with hysteroscopy, the sensitivity of the hystero-salpingogram was 74% and its specificity 60%. The false positive and false negative rates were 38.3% and 28.3% respectively. The most common findings on hysteroscopy were intrauterine adhesions (23.6%), followed by uterine septum (21.7%), and endometrial polyps (1.7%).[32] Hysteroscopic evaluation of the uterine cavity is much simpler than hysterosalpingography and should be the primary investigative procedure in habitual abortion.

Diagnostic office hysteroscopy also has application in cases of suspected proximal tubal obstruction. However, fluoroscopic attempts to diagnose and treat proximal tubal obstruction are also commonly performed. It is estimated that 15% of patients with tubal infertility have proximal obstruction. Sixteen (40%) of those obstructions shown on hysterosalpingography are false positives due to tubal spasm and mucous plugs. Under hysteroscopic guidance, visually directed insertion of tubal catheters allows the gynecologist to differentiate the patient having true proximal tubal occlusion from one having temporary occlusion.[3] The 5-mm flexible hysteroscope with a 2.2-mm working channel is particularly valuable for this application. The distal tip of the scope can be properly positioned with the thumb manipulator to allow exact placement of a catheter or probe into the oviduct. In five studies using hysteroscopic guidance combined with laparoscopy, 23 of 25 patients (92%) had successful cannulation of at least one fallopian tube, and 9 (39%) became pregnant within 3 to 7 months.[33] In summary, hysteroscopic cannulation of the fallopian tube is a safe diagnostic procedure that can be used to identify patients with true proximal tubal occlusion, as well as those with open tubes with mucous plugs and tubal spasm.[34]

During the past few years, flexible microendoscopes and accessory equipment have been developed, evaluated, and used for the safe transvaginal exploration of the entire length of the human fallopian tube.[34] Transuterine falloposcopy paves the way for atraumatic intraluminal adhesiolysis, removal of tubal ectopic pregnancies, and the performance of GIFT and ZIFT on an outpatient basis.[12]

GIFT by hysteroscopy as an alternative to the traditional GIFT by laparoscopy has recently been reported. Possati et al[35] performed hysteroscopic cannulation by a flexible catheter of the fallopian tubes for GIFT in 26 patients. They used a 4-mm 30° hysteroscope with CO_2 distention, and seven clinical pregnancies were established (25.9% per cycle). Patton et al[36] described a case of hysteroscopic retrograde directed fallopian tube catheterization and transfer of cryopreserved embryos. They used an office hysteroscope also with CO_2 distention. The tube was cannulated with a coaxial catheter, and an ongoing pregnancy was achieved with this transfer. Hysteroscopic GIFT, ZIFT, or TET are safe and simple alternatives to laparoscopic procedures. With the hysteroscopic procedures, general anesthesia is avoided, costs are lowered, and patient morbidity is greatly reduced.

Evaluating the uterine cavity before initiating an IVF cycle has been advocated. For reasons that are largely unknown, embryo implantation following transfer into the uterine cavity has the highest failure rate of any stage in the IVF procedure. It has been suggested that endometrial and structural uterine abnormalities are important factors in the causation of embryo replacement failure.[37] Shamma et al[38] performed an office hysteroscopy in 34 patients undergoing IVF who had normal hysterography. A total of 43% of patients had abnormal hysteroscopic findings, including small uterine septa, small submucous fibroids, uterine hypoplasia, and cervical ridges. Prospectively, the patients without a hysteroscopic abnormality achieved a significantly higher clinical pregnancy rate. Dicker et al[37] performed office hysteroscopy in 110 women with normal initial hysteroscopy who failed to conceive during three or more IVF-ET cycles. In 20 patients (18.2%) various abnormalities were detected, including endometrial hyperplasia, endometrial polyps, submucous fibroids, adhesions, and endometritis. Hyperplasia and polyps were correlated by histology. After correction of the uterine abnormalities, 13.9% clinical pregnancies per transfer were achieved in 43 subsequent IVF-ET cycles. Dicker et al[39] also found 29.9% uterine abnormalities among 284 women in whom diagnostic hysteroscopy was performed before IVF. Golan et al[29] diagnosed a 50% rate of intrauterine pathology (mainly intrauterine adhesions) with

hysteroscopy in 324 patients referred for hysterosalpingographic suspicion of an intrauterine abnormality or after a failed IVF-ET of good quality embryo. The conception rate was 22% after surgical treatment. Similarly, Kirshop et al[40] found a rate of 28% intrauterine abnormalities in 50 patients undergoing diagnostic hysteroscopy after two or more failed IVF-ET or GIFT cycles. One may consider obtaining a hysterosalpingogram to evaluate the uterus instead of office hysteroscopy. However, office hysteroscopy not only gives physicians a direct view of the endometrial cavity but also has the advantage of a decreased incidence of infection and discomfort compared with hysterosalpingography.[12] In view of the data, it is prudent that routine hysteroscopy be performed before entering an IVF program.

The pregnant patient

Hysteroscopy is rarely indicated in the pregnant patient. However, this technique should be considered in the following three clinical situations: to study an IUD in relation to early implantation, to perform embryoscopy, and to evaluate the "disturbed" pregnancy.

An intrauterine pregnancy can occur despite the presence of an IUD in 1% to 4% of patients. Because of the potential complication of septic abortion, preterm labor, increased incidence of spontaneous abortion, or possible teratogenic effect from copper-bearing devices, the IUD should be removed as soon as the pregnancy is diagnosed.[8,41] If abortion is indicated, the IUD should first be removed under hysteroscopic control before proceeding to suction curettage. In cases where pregnancy continuation is desired, the IUD can be removed, under direct vision, thus allowing the pregnancy to continue to term without complication.[8,41] Assaf et al[42] successfully removed an IUD with retracted tails in 46 of 52 pregnant women using a 7-mm hysteroscope with minimal CO_2 insufflation. The application of embryoscopy enables the physician to study the implantation site and early intrauterine fetal development. However, the technique is not simple or without hazard. Consequently, it should be considered experimental and limited to patients whose pregnancies are scheduled for termination by abortion. Hysteroscopy can be used to confirm a suspected complete abortion and help avoid unnecessary D&C. In cases of failed termination of pregnancy or difficult D&C, hysteroscopy can also help locate the implantation site and facilitate the D&C.[43] Hysteroscopy is also used for the confirmation of retained placental tissue in postpartum hemorrhage.[12]

Office hysteroscopy has been used to diagnose and treat tubal ectopic pregnancy. Marpeau et al[44] performed diagnostic hysteroscopy in 60 patients with suspected ectopic pregnancy when viable uterine pregnancy had been ruled out. The sensitivity of hysteroscopy for the diagnosis of ectopic pregnancy was 100% with a specificity of 95%. Kullander and Maltau[45] reported two cases of tubal pregnancy successfully treated with hysteroscopic tubal instillation of prostaglandin F2-alpha using a Hamou hysteroscope and CO_2 insufflation.

Hysteroscopy can also be useful in assessing patients with a suspected interstitial pregnancy. Interstitial pregnancy is known to be rare, with an incidence between 1 in 2500 and 1 in 5000 live births. Even with laparoscopy and ultrasound, the diagnosis is sometimes difficult to establish. Reported ultrasonic features include an eccentrically located gestational sac surrounded by an asymmetric myometrial mantle and a separate empty uterine cavity. Hysteroscopic conservative management may be feasible in the case of an early, unruptured interstitial pregnancy, allowing preservation of pelvic organs and future fertility. Kabukoba and de Courcy-Wheeler[46] reported two cases in which the diagnosis of interstitial pregnancy was uncertain. In the first case, an intrauterine pregnancy was confirmed at 11 weeks using a 5-mm hysteroscope and CO_2 distention. This patient had an uneventful pregnancy and a normal delivery at term. In the second patient, hysteroscopy demonstrated an empty uterus at 10 weeks. A subsequent laparotomy confirmed the diagnosis of interstitial pregnancy. Meyer and Mitchell[47] reported a case of suspected interstitial pregnancy that was confirmed by laparoscopy and hysteroscopy. The pregnancy was successfully treated by laparoscopically guided hysteroscopic removal of the products of conception. Similarly, Budnick et al[48] reported a case in which hysteroscopy was performed at 8 weeks that revealed a massively dilated tubal ostium with diffuse gestational tissue in the interstitial portion of the tube. The ectopic pregnancy was successfully treated with curettage of the dilated interstitial portion of the tube under laparoscopic visualization. Goldenberg et al[49] used local methotrexate administration through hysteroscopic vision to successfully treat a 7-week cornual pregnancy diagnosed by ultrasound. The hysteroscopy was performed under local anesthesia with an 8-mm double-channel operative hysteroscope. In summary, hysteroscopy can be an important tool in the diagnosis and management of selected cases of tubal or interstitial ectopic pregnancy.

Evaluation of the cervical canal, internal cervical os, and uterine cavity in patients with a history of habitual abortion, previous surgical procedures, or cervical dysplasia

Panoramic diagnostic office hysteroscopy is an ideal method for examining the endocervical canal for evidence of polyps or vascular changes. It has no application in the study of the patient with either an incompetent cervix or frank carcinoma of the cervix. Hamou[50] developed and popularized the microcolpohysteroscope for evaluation of patients suspected of having cervical pathology. This unique endoscope has a double optical system that allows not only for panoramic hysteroscopic examination of the uterine cavity and cervix but also a contact mode for the examination of the cervical portio and endocervical canal in patients suspected of having cervical intraepithelial neoplasia. In the contact mode, magnification can be adjusted to $20\times$, $60\times$, or $150\times$ to allow for dramatic in vivo magnification of the cells at the squamo-columnar junction. As is the case with standard colposcopy, tissue from suspicious lesions can be obtained for biopsy under direct vision to allow for histologic diagnostic confirmation. Also, the finer differentiation of the ectocervical abnormalities may influence management by identification of the upper limit of the transformation zone that could not be seen with the colposcope. This, in turn, can subsequently reduce the number or size of necessary cone biopsies.[12]

Diagnostic hysteroscopy, either along with or in place of hysterosalpingography, can be a most valuable tool in assessing uterine defects in patients who have undergone procedures such as myomectomies, hysterotomies, cesarean sections, and metroplasties.

Staging of patients with suspected carcinoma of the uterus

In the evaluation and staging of patients with suspected uterine cancer, hysteroscopy has no equal.[51-53] Hysteroscopy can clearly display the appearance of the cancer and its involvement of the lower uterine segment and cervix. In one study, convincing evidence of the efficacy of hysteroscopy has been obtained from the histologic examination of the uterus after hysterectomy in 80 patients with endometrial carcinoma. Hysteroscopy failed to detect the distal border of the cancer correctly in only 3% of patients. Not surprisingly, in this small number of patients' uteri, the malignant growth had reached the cervix through submucosal extension within the myometrium rather than by surface endometrial extension.[51] Taddei et al[54] performed hysteroscopic examination of the endometrial cavity and the cervical canal in 235 cases of primary endometrial adenocarcinoma before hysterectomy. They concluded that the hysteroscope played an important role in the diagnosis of an endometrial cancer and allowed a quite precise evaluation of the tumor's clinical stage (stage I vs. stage II), but it was unable to determine, based on the tumor's intrauterine dimensions, the degree of myometrial invasion. The use of hysteroscopy for examining patients with endometrial carcinoma has been questioned because of concerns regarding the risk of spreading cancer through the fallopian tubes into the abdominal cavity. Romano et al[55] reported a case of clinical stage IA grade 2 endometrial adenocarcinoma diagnosed by hysteroscopy and directed biopsies. Surgical staging revealed positive cytology suggesting that endometrial irrigation during hysteroscopy could have been the means of entry of malignant cells into the peritoneal cavity. However, medical centers using hysterosalpingography—which allows for similar spill into the peritoneal cavity, as does hysteroscopy—have demonstrated no increased risk of intraabdominal spread of endometrial carcinoma.[56] Tanizawa et al[57] reviewed 1040 hysteroscopies performed in the management of endometrial cancer. Compared with a group of 2641 women with endometrial cancer who did not have hysteroscopy before operation, they found that hysteroscopy had no effect on cytologic malignancy in the peritoneal cavity. Likewise, Sugimoto[52] diagnosed 33 cases of endometrial cancer among 4000 hysteroscopic examinations and found no extrauterine implants at laparoscopy done a few weeks later. Ranta et al[62] demonstrated that hysteroscopy leads to dissemination of endometrial cells in the peritoneal fluid but less frequently than chromotubation. Despite those reassuring reports, controversy remains whether dissemination of cells in cases of endometrial cancer is detrimental to the patient.[12] The advantages of hysteroscopy acquire even more importance in light of the comparable disadvantages of fractional curettage. The main disadvantage of curettage is the possibility of going beyond the canal and obtaining material from the isthmus and uterine cavity that is considered to be endocervical.

Another, although less frequent, oncologic use of hysteroscopy is the follow-up of any nonsurgical treatment of endometrial carcinoma. Hysteroscopy allows for a "second look" in patients with advanced carcinomas that cannot be surgically extirpated and that have been treated with radiation therapy. Hysteroscopy has also been useful in extracting radium capsules that were "lost" in the uterine cavity.

Routine office hysteroscopy to increase detection of endometrial carcinoma is not recommended at this point. Iossa et al[18] reviewed 2007 incidents of office hysteroscopy and found that detecting one cancer resulted in 419, 148, 130, 48, and 12 unnecessary hysteroscopies in women younger than age 45, 45-49, 50-54, 55-64, or older than 64, respectively. Routine hysteroscopy should therefore be carefully considered in selected patients, at least under age 45.

ATTEMPTS AT TUBAL OCCLUSION TO EFFECT STERILIZATION

Many hysteroscopic techniques of sterilization have received clinical evaluation under various research protocols.[58,59] Hysteroscopically directed transcervical sterilization procedures can be divided into three categories based on the mechanism of tubal occlusion: destruction of the interstitial portion of the oviduct by thermal energy (electrocoagulation or cryosurgery);[60] injection techniques to deliver sclerosing substances or tissue adhesives such as quinacrine gelatine, resorcinol, formaldehyde, and methylcyanoacrylate (Crazy Glue);[33] and mechanical occlusive devices or plugs to block the oviduct such as the uterotubal junction device, the P-block plug, the silicone rubber device, the Popp-claw device, or a uterotubal ceramic plug.[3,12,59] Initial enthusiasm regarding hysteroscopically directed tubal coagulation vanished after a multicenter study reported many major complications including tubal and cornual ectopic pregnancies, excessive uterine bleeding and perforation, and acute and prolonged endometritis with pain, bleeding, fever, and bowel damage with resultant peritonitis.[60] The majority of injection techniques using caustic chemicals does not require use of hysteroscopy. Methylcyanoacrylate and quinacrine have received the greatest clinical investigation.[3,59] Oviductal occlusion with preformed blocking devices has been tried but with little clinical success. Brundin[61]

reported a 10-year experience with the P-block. The gross Pearl Index was 5, due to rejection of the device on either one or both sides. The corresponding value for intact P-blocks in situ was 0.3. On the other hand, hysteroscopic application of a formed-in-place Silastic oviductal plug has been shown to be both safe and effective in expanded clinical trials.[3,59] During an FDA-approved clinical investigation spanning 6 years, more than 2000 American women underwent this unique sterilization procedure. The majority of procedures was performed in an office setting using a 4.0 -mm rigid telescope housed in a 70-mm operative sheath having a 7 French operative channel. Thirty-two percent dextran (Hyskon) was used for uterine distention. The majority of patients received a paracervical block consisting of 12 ml of 1% lidocaine hydrochloride (Xylocaine) to allow for the length of the procedure, which extended anywhere from 20 to 45 minutes. During a 5-minute period and under direct visual control, liquid Silastic material flowed through a catheter into the oviduct, curing in place to occlude the tubal lumen. In those patients who had successful bilateral plug placement (confirmed by radiologic flat plate examination of the pelvis) the pregnancy rate was less than 1%. Bilateral plug placement was possible in 13% of the patient population. Reasons for a "failed" procedure included tubal spasm, poor intrauterine visualization, unusual anatomic factors, intravasation of silicone, and technical difficulties with the Silastic material and catheters.

Contraindications to Office Hysteroscopy

The indications for office hysteroscopy are many; absolute contraindications to performing the procedure are few (see box). Perhaps the most important among them would be inadequate operator experience and/or inappropriate or ineffectual instrumentation. "Watch one, do one, teach one" is no longer an accepted standard of practice. Physicians who wish to perform diagnostic office hysteroscopy must undergo a period of formal training.[8] To minimize patient complaints of pelvic pain and the occasional vasovagal reaction,

---

Contraindications for office hysteroscopy

Absolute contraindications

Inadequate operator experience
Inadequate instrumentation
Uncooperative patient
Cervical cancer
Acute pelvic inflammatory disease

Relative contraindications

Cervicitis and/or vaginitis
Pregnancy
Active uterine bleeding
Severe cervical stenosis
Severe cardiorespiratory disease and/or metabolic acidosis

physicians must be able to carry on a comfortable and reassuring dialogue with their patient during the short diagnostic procedure. If possible, the examination should be performed under video control to allow the patient to be an active participant in the procedure. The video image can be useful as a source both of patient distraction and education. When necessary, pre-procedure sedation or analgesia should be offered. Meticulous technique and slow, careful insertion of the telescope are required to avoid undesirable bleeding from the endocervical canal and endometrium.

Hysteroscopy should not be performed in cases of suspected pelvic inflammatory disease except when a lost IUD is thought to be responsible. In these rare cases, quick hysteroscopic examination and IUD removal are justifiable after appropriate antibiotic therapy has been initiated.

Although ascending infection is a rare complication of office diagnostic hysteroscopy, it is best to delay the hysteroscopic examination in patients who have clear evidence of cervicitis or vaginitis until the condition has been adequately treated. The extremely low incidence of such ascending infection should not be allowed to negatively affect good sterile technique and proper antiseptic cleansing of the vagina and cervix before insertion of the hysteroscope.

Pregnancy is a relative contraindication to hysteroscopy. Despite the safety afforded by properly calibrated low-flow CO_2 hysteroflators, the theoretic possibility of a CO_2 embolus is a concern. Should hysteroscopic examination of the pregnant patient become absolutely necessary, CO_2 flow rates should be limited to 30 cc/minute and intrauterine pressures should not exceed 40 to 50 mm Hg. Such precautions will minimize the possibilities of carbon dioxide embolization, placental separation, and retroplacental bleeding.[41]

Unlike cases of suspected endometrial cancer, cervical cancer is a contraindication to office diagnostic hysteroscopy.[2,8] No diagnostic or therapeutic benefit is derived from such an examination, and the increased risk of bleeding or cervical laceration from such an endeavor is unwarranted.

Uterine bleeding is sometimes offered as a contraindication to diagnostic office hysteroscopy. If the bleeding is thought to be menstrual in nature, and is not life-threatening, it is far more appropriate to delay the hysteroscopic examination until some time during the early proliferative phase of the patient's menstrual cycle. In cases of anovulatory bleeding, the procedure is best done when the patient is not actively bleeding. When such delay is not possible or inappropriate, a successful examination is possible even in patients who are actively bleeding.[50] Although the very experienced operator may be able to satisfactorily employ CO_2 distention of the cavity in these cases, it is more prudent to consider a high-viscosity distention medium (32% dextran [Hyskon]) or to employ low-viscosity liquids with continuous-flow technology. Suction curettage with a small curette can often free the uterine cavity of blood and clots and allow adequate visualization.[7] It is of utmost importance not to advance the hysteroscope in a clouded or bloody field. If the scope is advanced in such a situation, uterine perforation is likely.

In rare circumstances, the scope and sheath will not pass easily through the cervical canal into the uterine cavity. This occurrence is more likely with rigid hysteroscopes, and in such cases the risks of cervical laceration, uterine perforation, and unacceptable patient discomfort are significant. Bimanual examination is critical to determine the uterine position before inserting a uterine sound or cervical dilator. Gentle probing of the ectocervix with lacrimal duct dilators will often allow a narrow ectocervical opening into which a narrow rigid or flexible hysteroscope can be inserted. Gentle insertion of the hysteroscope, under direct visualization, will avoid the creation of a false channel. When such techniques are employed, most nulliparous and postmenopausal cervices can be negotiated. The most difficult patient to examine is one who has cervical scarring as a result of a cervical conization procedure, especially if she has been exposed to diethylstilbestrol in utero. When reasonable attempts at cervical dilatation and telescope insertion are thwarted, the procedure should be terminated and rescheduled for an outpatient surgical setting where general anesthesia is available.

A confused, uncooperative, and anxious patient makes an office diagnostic hysteroscopic procedure all but impossible. Often, such a patient is elderly and possesses a narrow introitus, atrophic vagina, and atrophic cervix with a pinpoint cervical os. These anatomic limitations make the patient a better candidate for the operating room and general anesthesia.

Severe cardiorespiratory disease and/or metabolic acidosis are relative contraindications to office hysteroscopy. However, a short office diagnostic procedure, requiring no general anesthesia and little or no local anesthesia, can be an attractive alternative to the more complex in-hospital procedure.

CONCLUSION

Hysteroscopy can be learned and practiced by most gynecologists; however, it does require specialized training. Office hysteroscopy has been shown to be safe and useful in the diagnosis and management of patients with many gynecologic problems. Hysteroscopic procedures carry little risk and are both cost and time effective. An increasing number of didactic and hands-on educational programs enable all interested physicians to learn this technique. After some initial experience with patients asleep in the operating room, the physician should strive to bring this innovative technology into the office, particularly for the large number of patients with abnormal uterine bleeding. In all of the conditions discussed in this chapter, diagnostic office hysteroscopy, when performed early in the evaluation plan, will allow for the identification of significant abnormalities that might otherwise go undiagnosed.

REFERENCES

1. Pantaleoni D: On endoscopic examination of the cavity of the womb, *Med Press Circ* 8:26, 1869.

2. Sugimoto O: *Diagnostic and therapeutic hysteroscopy,* Tokyo, 1978, Igakushoin.
3. Cooper JM, Houck RM: The incidence of intrauterine abnormalities found at hysteroscopic sterilization, *J Reprod Med* 28:659, 1983.
4. Gimpelson RJ, Rappold HD: A comparative study between panoramic hysteroscopy with directed biopsies and dilatation and curettage, *Am J Obstet Gynecol* 158:489, 1988.
5. Loffer FD: Hysteroscopy with selective endometrial sampling compared with D&C for abnormal uterine bleeding: the value of a negative hysteroscopic view, *Obstet Gynecol* 73:16-20, 1989.
6. Burnett JE: Hysteroscopy-controlled curettage for endometrial polyps, *Obstet Gynecol* 24:621, 1964.
7. Gimpelson RJ: Office hysteroscopy, *Clin Obstet Gynecol* 35(2):270, 1992.
8. Taylor PJ and Gordon AG: *Practical hysteroscopy* 24 London, 1983, Blackwell Scientific Publications Inc.
9. Englund S, Ingelman-Sundberg A, Westin B: Hysteroscopy in diagnosis and treatment of uterine bleeding, *Gynaecologia* 143:217, 1957.
10. Taylor PJ, Cumming DC: Hysteroscopy in 100 patients, *Fertil Steril,* 31:301, 1979.
11. ACOG Technical Bulletin No. 191, April 1994: Hysteroscopy, *Int J Gynecol Obstet* 45:175, 1994.
12. Finikiotos G: Hysteroscopy: a review, *Obstet Gynecol Surv* 49(4):273, 1994.
13. Vercellini P et al: Abnormal uterine bleeding associated with iron deficiency anemia: etiology and role of hysteroscopy, *J Reprod Med* 38(7):502, 1993.
14. Fedele L et al: Transvaginal ultrasonography versus hysteroscopy in the diagnosis of uterine submucous myomas, *Obstet Gynecol* 77:745, 1991.
15. Cicinelli E et al: Transabdominal sonohysterography, transvaginal sonography, and hysteroscopy in the evaluation of submucous myomas, *Obstet Gynecol,* 85:42, 1995.
16. Lei ZW, Xie L: Hysteroscopic findings in women with IUD-induced menorrhagia, *Int J Gynecol Obstet,* 42:173, 1993.
17. Coeman D et al: Hysteroscopic findings in patients with a cervical polyp, *Am J Obstet Gynecol* 169:1563, 1993.
18. Iossa A et al: Hysteroscopy and endometrial cancer diagnosis: a review of 2007 consecutive examinations in self-referred patients, *Tumori* 77:479, 1991.
19. Altaras MM et al: Microhysteroscopy and endometrial biopsy results following failed diagnostic dilatation and curettage in women with postmenopausal bleeding *Int J Gynecol Obstet* 42:255, 1993.
20. Cacciatore B et al: Transvaginal sonography and hysteroscopy in postmenopausal bleeding, *Acta Obstet Gynecol Scand* 73:413, 1994.
21. Townsend DE et al: Diagnostic and operative hysteroscopy in the management of persistent postmenopausal bleeding, *Obstet Gynecol* 82:419, 1993.
22. Downes E, Al-Azzawi F: The predictive value of outpatient hysteroscopy in a menopause clinic, *Br J Obstet Gynaecol* 100:1148, 1993.
23. Valle RF, Freeman DW: Hysteroscopy in the localization and removal of intrauterine devices with "missing" strings, *Contraception* 11:161, 1975.
24. Marcus SF et al: Endometrial ossification: a cause of secondary infertility. Report of two cases, *Am J Obstet Gynecol* 170(5):1381, 1994.
25. Borgatta L, Barad D: Prolonged retention of laminaria fragments: an unusual complication of laminaria usage, *Obstet Gynecol* 78:988, 1991.
26. Romano F et al: Sonohysterography versus hysteroscopy for diagnosing endouterine abnormalities in fertile women, *Int J Gynecol Obstet,* 45:253, 1994.
27. Rosenfeld DL: A study of hysteroscopy as an adjunct to laparoscopy in the evaluation of the infertile woman. In Phillips JM, Ed: *Endoscopy in gynecology,* Downey, Calif., 1977, American Association of Gynecologic Laparoscopists.
28. Sciarra JJ, Valle RF: Hysteroscopy: A clinical experience with 320 patients, *Am J Obstet Gynecol* 127:340, 1977.
29. Golan A et al: Diagnostic hysteroscopy: its value in an in-vitro fertilization/embryo transfer unit, *Hum Reprod* 7(10):1433, 1992.
30. March CM, Israel R, March AD: Hysteroscopic management of intrauterine adhesions, *Am J Obstet Gynecol,* 130:653, 1978.
31. DeCherney AH et al: Resectoscopic management of mullerian fusion defects, *Fertil Steril* 45:726, 1987.
32. Raziel A et al: Investigation of the uterine cavity in recurrent aborters, *Fertil Steril,* 62(5):1080, 1994.
33. Flood JT, Grow DR: Transcervical tubal cannulation: a review, *Obstet Gynecol Surv* 48(11):768, 1993.
34. Kerin JF, Surrey ES: Tubal surgery from the inside out: falloposcopy and balloon tuboplasty, *Clin Obstet Gynecol* 35(2):299, 1992.
35. Possati G et al: Gamete intrafallopian transfer by hysteroscopy as an alternative treatment for infertility, *Fertil Steril* 56:496, 1991.
36. Patton PE, Hickok LR, Wolf DP: Successful hysteroscopic cannulation and tubal transfer of cryopreserved embryos, *Fertil Steril* 55(3):640, 1991.
37. Dicker D et al: The value of repeat hysteroscopic evaluation in patients with failed in vitro fertilization transfer cycles, *Fertil Steril* 58(4):833, 1992.
38. Shamma FN et al: The role of office hysteroscopy in in-vitro fertilization, *Fertil Steril* 58(6):1237, 1992.
39. Dicker D et al: The value of hysteroscopy in elderly women prior to in vitro fertilization-embryo transfer (IVF-ET): a comparative study, *J In Vitro Fert Embryo Transf* 7(5):267, 1990.
40. Kirshop R et al: The role of hysteroscopy in patients having failed IVF/GIFT transfer cycles, *Aust N Z J Obstet Gynaecol* 31(3):263, 1991.
41. Gallinat A: Hysteroscopy in early pregnancy. In Siegler AM, Ed: *Hysteroscopy principles and management,* Philadelphia, 1964, J.P. Lippincott.
42. Assaf A et al: Removal of intrauterine devices with missing tails during early pregnancy, *Contraception* 45:541, 1992.
43. Valle RF, Sabbagha RE: Management of first trimester pregnancy termination failure, *Obstet Gynecol* 55:625, 1980.
44. Marpeau L et al: Hysteroscopic diagnosis of ectopic pregnancy, *Eur J Obstet Gynecol Reprod Biol* 46(1):31, 1992.
45. Kullander S, Maltau JM: Treatment of unruptured tubal pregnancy by an hysteroscopic procedure, *Acta Obstet Gynecol Scand* 70:247, 1991.
46. Kabukoba JJ, de Courcy-Wheeler RHB: Hysteroscopy in the diagnosis of suspected interstitial pregnancy, *Int J Gynecol Obstet* 37:121, 1992.
47. Meyer WR, Mitchell DE: Hysteroscopic removal of an interstitial ectopic gestation, *J Reprod Med* 34(11), 1989.
48. Budnick SJ et al: Conservative management of interstitial pregnancy, *Obstet Gynecol Surv* 48(10):694, 1993.
49. Goldenberg M et al: Treatment of interstitial pregnancy with methotrexate via hysteroscopy, *Fertil Steril* 58(6):1234, 1992.
50. Hamou J: Microhysteroscopy: a new procedure and its original applications in gynecology, *J Reprod Med* 26:375, 1981.
51. Joelsson I: Hysteroscopy in delineating the intrauterine extent of endometrial cancer. In Seigler AM, Ed: *Hysteroscopy principles and management,* Philadelphia, 1982, J.B. Lippincott.
52. Sugimoto O: Hysteroscopic diagnosis of endometrial cancer, *Am J Obstet Gynecol* 121:109, 1975.
53. Valle RF: Hysteroscopic evaluation of patients with abnormal uterine bleeding, *Surg Gynecol Obstet* 153:521, 1982.
54. Taddei GL et al: Can hysteroscopic evaluation of endometrial carcinoma influence therapeutic treatment? *Ann N Y Acad Sci* 734:482, 1994.
55. Romano S et al: Case report: retrograde seeding of endometrial carcinoma during hysteroscopy, *Gynecol Oncol* 44:116, 1992.
56. Norman O: Hysterography in cancer of the corpus of the uterus, *Acta Radiol Suppl* 79, 1950.

57. Tanizawa O, Miyake A, Sugimoto O: Re-evaluation of hysteroscopy in the diagnosis of uterine endometrial cancer, *Nippon Sanka Fujinka Gakkai Zasshi* 43(6):622, 1991.
58. Cooper JM: Hysteroscopic sterilization, *Clin Obstet Gynecol* 35:282, 1992.
59. Cooper JM: Hysteroscopic sterilization. In Corson SL, Ed: *Fertility control,* Boston, 1985, Little, Brown & Co.
60. Darabi KF, Richart RH: Collaborative study on hysteroscopic sterilization procedures, Preliminary report, *Obstet Gynecol* 49:48, 1977.
61. Brundin J: Transcervical sterilization in the human female by hysteroscopic application of hydrogelic occlusive devices into the intramural parts of the fallopian tubes: 10 years experience of the P-block, *Eur J Obstet Gynecol Reprod Biol* 39(1):41, 1991.
62. Ranta H et al: Dissemination of endometrial cells during carbon dioxide hysteroscopy and chromotubation among infertile patients, *Fertil Steril* 53:751, 1990.

Chapter 3

SELECTING THE PROPER EQUIPMENT FOR OFFICE RIGID HYSTEROSCOPY

Keith B. Isaacson

As with all endoscopic procedures, a variety of equipment is available to perform office hysteroscopy. Given the constant advances in technology, one is always concerned that no matter what is purchased, a new and better product will soon be on the market. Despite this fear, one should be encouraged to know that it is not unusual to own hysteroscopic equipment for many years that remains functional and practical.

However, a physician must consider several factors before purchasing the necessary equipment to perform office hysteroscopy. Examples of these factors include the age and parity of patients who are to be evaluated, the necessity of photo-documentation, the availability of sterilization facilities, and the local reimbursement standard.

Office hysteroscopy can be performed with a minimal amount of equipment: a hysteroscope, a fiber optic cable, and a light source. The average cost for this equipment will range from $7500 to $10,000. At the other end of the spectrum, an elaborate teaching unit can consist of diagnostic and operative hysteroscopes (3.5 to 5.5 mm), a 300 W light source, a digitized camera, a high-resolution monitor, a video printer, a video recorder, a slidemaker, and a video procedures cart. All of this equipment together will cost $25,000 to $30,000. This chapter will review all of the available equipment for office hysteroscopy to help physicians decide what is the best equipment to purchase for their particular practice.

HYSTEROSCOPES

The goal of office hysteroscopy is to adequately visualize the entire endometrial cavity with as little patient discomfort

as possible. The majority of discomfort results from cervical dilatation and manipulation with little discomfort arising from uterine distention. Therefore the office hysteroscope should have the smallest outer diameter (O.D.) possible that will provide adequate visualization of the entire endometrial cavity. Office hysteroscopes range in size from 3 to 5.5 mm and are available with rigid or flexible optical systems. In addition, a rigid 5.5-mm system has recently become available with continuous-flow capabilities.

Rigid hysteroscopes

All hysteroscopes contain three vital components: a transmitting lens system to bring light into the uterine cavity, a transmitting lens system to carry the reflected light from the cavity to the eyepiece, and a magnifying eyepiece.[1] In the rigid hysteroscopes all three components are surrounded by a steel skin.

The traditional lens system comprised a series of glass lenses separated by air throughout a 35-mm shaft. Because glass will transmit light more efficiently than air, the newer systems transmit light through glass rods with very little (Hopkins system) or no (Gradient Index lens system) interspersed air (Fig. 3-1).

Diagnostic rigid hysteroscopes are available with a 3 mm, 4 mm, or 5 mm O.D. These scopes require a sheath that is at least 0.3 mm larger than the scope (3.3 mm, 4.3 mm, 5.3 mm). As one would expect, the larger the O.D. of the hysteroscope the greater the amount of light that is transmitted into and out of the uterine cavity. If necessary, one can overcome the limited amount of light transmitted through the smaller scopes by increasing the intensity of the

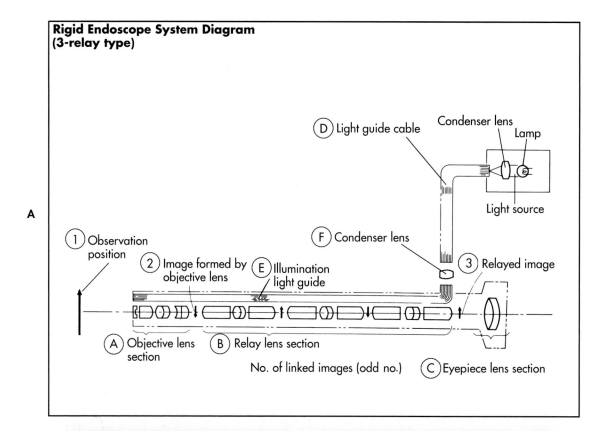

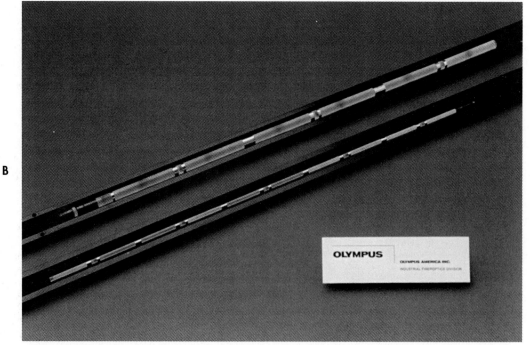

Fig. 3-1. Rigid hysteroscope system. **A,** Diagram of a rigid hysteroscope using the glass rod-lens system that relays the image to the eyepiece section. (Courtesy Storz, Boston, Mass.) **B,** Photograph of the rigid hysteroscope rod-lens system. (Courtesy Olympus America, Inc, Industrial Fiberoptics Division, Lake Success, NY.)

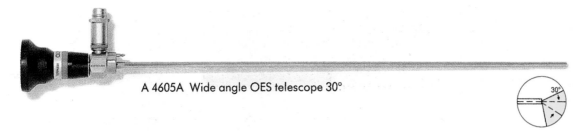

A 4605A Wide angle OES telescope 30°

Fig. 3-2. 30° Rigid hysteroscope. Terminal objective of 30° is most useful in anteflexed or retroflexed uteri. (Courtesy Olympus America, Inc, Industrial Fiberoptics Division, Lake Success, NY.)

light source. Most rigid hysteroscopes come at a length of 35 cm; however, shorter 3-mm O.D. pediatric cystoscopes are available for unusual circumstances.

The terminal objective is available at angles of 0°, 12°, 30°, 70°, and 90°. Of these, the 30° lens is the most convenient to use for office diagnostic hysteroscopy (Fig. 3-2). The 0° or 12° lens is used for midpositioned uteri; the 30° lens is more appropriate with anteflexed and retroflexed uteri. The actual field of view is dependent not only on the angle of the terminal objective but also on the distending media. The view is wider with CO_2 than with aqueous distention because of its larger refractive index.

A hysteroscopic sheath is necessary for rigid panoramic hysteroscopy to allow distention media to flow into the uterine cavity. The sheath consists of a hollow stainless steel tube that has a proximal connecting port. Manufacturers of hysteroscopes each use a unique locking system, which provides a tight seal to prevent leakage of distending media. The distal end of the sheath should be flush with the hysteroscope so as not to obstruct the view of the uterine cavity. The O.D. of the diagnostic hysteroscopic sheath, as mentioned, is approximately 0.3 to 1 mm larger than the hysteroscope.

Operative hysteroscopic sheaths are available that until recently required an O.D. of 7.5 to 8.5 mm. These sheaths are available in single channel or multichannel configurations, which will allow the passage of flexible and semirigid instruments such as scissors and biopsy forceps. It is my view that hysteroscopy requiring significant cervical dilatation to allow the passage of an 8-mm instrument should be done only in the operating room and not the office. Cervical dilatation places the patient at greater risk of uterine perforation, significant vasovagal reactions, and morbidity from the pain of cervical dilatation. All office procedures should be done with hysteroscopes that have an O.D. of 5.5 mm or less.

Until recently, all office rigid hysteroscopies had to be done in the early proliferative phase and with little uterine bleeding to visualize the uterine cavity. This limitation reduces the flexibility of office hysteroscopy and occasionally requires hormonal suppression in patients with poly-

menorrhea. Because instrumentation with a single outer sheath does not allow adequate fluid outflow, any bleeding will cloud the view. With CO_2 distention, mucus and blood will often obstruct visualization of the cavity. Small O.D. (5.5. mm) continuous-flow hysteroscopic systems have been available only since the spring of 1994. The continuous flow system consists of a single sheath with two channels: a large channel in which a 3-mm 30° rigid hysteroscope is placed and an operative channel large enough to pass 1.6-mm semirigid and flexible instruments (Fig. 3-3). This design allows fluid to be instilled into the channel around the hysteroscope and into the cavity and provides outflow through the operative channel in which instruments are passed. The continuous-flow system also provides excellent clarity even with moderate uterine bleeding. This system is ideal for any patient who is bleeding and requires removal of tissue for biopsy.

There is little debate that rigid hysteroscopy, using a 3- or 4-mm hysteroscope, provides the optics and light for excellent visualization of the uterine cavity. However, a distinct disadvantage to office rigid hysteroscopy is pa-tient discomfort. A rigid hysteroscope is a straight, inflexible metal instrument. It must be inserted through the cervix and into the uterine cavity, which most often is a curved path (Fig. 3-4). As a result, a tenaculum must be placed on the cervix, and the cervix and uterus must be pulled toward the operator to straighten the canal and allow passage of the hysteroscope (Fig. 3-5). This technique can produce moderate to severe discomfort. It most often necessitates the placement of a paracervical block, which will ordinarily add 10 to 15 minutes to the procedure. In addition, the passage of a straight, rigid instrument through a curved canal increases the risk of uterine perforation and significant vasovagal reactions. These two factors have influenced the growth of office flexible hysteroscopy. The flexible hysteroscope, with its distal end capable of bending up to 110°, can be guided through the endocervical canal into the endometrial cavity using a no-touch technique without the placement of a cervical tenaculum or paracervical block (Fig. 3-6). With the high-quality optics available in flexible hysteroscopes, office flexible hysteroscopy can

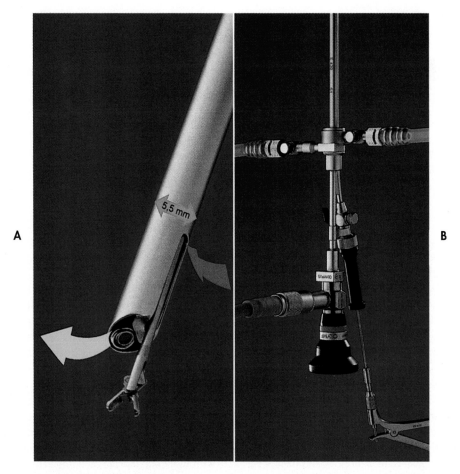

Fig. 3-3. Continuous-flow office hysteroscope. A 5.5-mm continuous-flow system in which the fluid is instilled through the inner channel and returns through the operative channel. **A,** The operative end of the 5.5-mm continuous-flow system. **B,** The inflow and outflow connections for the 5.5-mm continuous-flow system. (Courtesy Olympus America, Inc, Medical Instruments Division, Lake Success, NY.)

be performed with the equivalent clarity of rigid hysteroscopy. In addition, flexible hysteroscopy is associated with a decreased risk of uterine perforation and less discomfort than is rigid hysteroscopy. Continuous-flow hysteroscopes, however, are currently available only with rigid sheaths.

Light sources. Light sources available for office hysteroscopy include a 150 to 250 W tungsten/iodine vapor, a 150 to 250 W halogen-quartz incandescent lamp, a 150 to 300 W mercury-halide lamp, or a 175 to 300 W xenon vapor arc lamp.[2] The color of the light emitted depends on the temperature of the source. The temperature is measured in degrees Kelvin (K°). Light sources with higher K° emit a higher-frequency blue light, which results in a brighter, more accurate image. Although the tungsten/iodine vapor and the halogen-quartz lamps (2800 to 3400 K°) are generally less expensive, their light does not contain the high-quality blue light produced by the mercury-halide or xenon lights (5600 to 6600 K°). The bulb life of the mercury-halide

arc lamp is approximately 250 hours, and the bulb life of the xenon lamp is approximately 1000 hours.

The light source generates a great deal of heat and must be cooled by a fan within the light source. The heat from the light is dissipated as the light travels through the fiberoptic light cables. The light emitted from the light cables is therefore referred to as "cold light."

The amount of light needed for office hysteroscopy will depend on the type of laparoscope used, the distention medium, and the presence or absence of uterine bleeding or discharge, as well as the use of beam splitters, video couplers, and cameras. If a rigid 3- or 4-mm hysteroscope or a flexible 4.9-mm hysteroscope is being used, then a 150 to 175 W halogen, xenon, or mercury-halide light source is usually sufficient (Fig. 3-7). Because of the reduced number of light bundles available in the flexible 3.6-mm hysteroscope, a 175 to 300 W light source is necessary (Fig. 3-8). Bleeding or mucous discharge will reflect less light through the hysteroscope than a tan to white atrophic endometrium

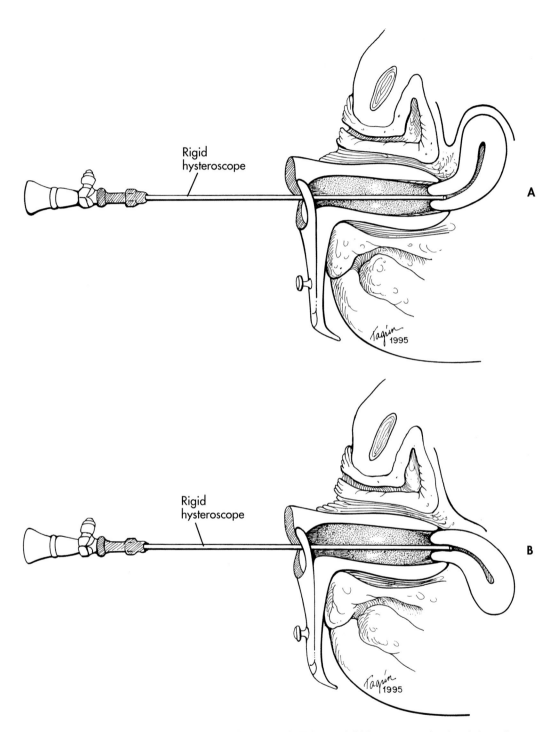

Fig. 3-4. Rigid hysteroscope placement in uterus. **A,** When a rigid hysteroscope is placed through the cervical canal of an anteflexed uterus, the posterior endometrial wall will be encountered. **B,** When a rigid hysteroscope is placed through the cervical canal of a retroflexed uterus, the anterior endometrial wall will be encountered.

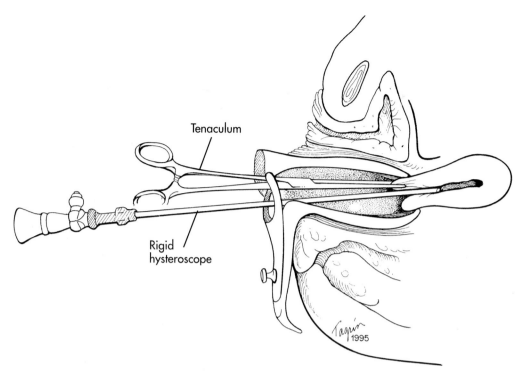

Fig. 3-5. Proper placement of rigid hysteroscope. A tenaculum is placed on the anterior lip of the cervix. The cervix is pulled toward the operator to straighten the uterine canal to allow insertion of a rigid hysteroscope.

will. Video and photo apparatuses will also reduce the light transmitted and therefore necessitate the 175 to 300 W light source.

Fiberoptic cables, composed of multiple coaxial quartz fibers, are necessary to transmit the light from the light source to the hysteroscope. The individual light fibers are 6 to 25 μm in diameter and consist of an inner quartz core surrounded by a nonrefractive outer sheath. The light will exit the distal end of the fiber after many internal refractions.

In a light cable, incoherent bundles are manufactured by randomly packing multiple fibers together with filler material. Incoherent cables will lose approximately 30% of the light to heat transmission. Cables in which the fibers are arranged in oriented bundles are referred to as coherent cables. This arrangement produces a true image when the bundles are fused and focused at the distal end of the cable. Coherent cables are much more expensive than incoherent cables and are used exclusively in flexible hysteroscopes.

Fiberoptic light cables, although fragile, will last indefinitely if properly maintained. Damage to the fiber bundles can be assessed by shining the light on a flat surface. Broken fibers show up as black dots. If more than 25% of the fibers are damaged, the cable should be replaced.

Video display

It is reasonable for physicians who are just beginning to perform office hysteroscopy to use only the minimal equip-

ment necessary: the hysteroscope, light source, and light cable. This system can be purchased for $3500 to $6000 depending on whether a rigid or flexible system is chosen. This initial investment will be sufficient to allow physicians to decide whether they have appropriate patient volume to justify a video system. The advantages of the video system include surgeon comfort, image magnification, patient and assistant viewing, and video documentation. The working lengths of the hysteroscopes range from 16 to 30 cm; therefore, the surgeon must get very close to the patient to look through the scope. Using video, the surgeon can be at a more comfortable distance from the patient. We ask all of our patients whether they would like to observe the hysteroscopy, and we will explain our findings as we see them. Approximately 70% of the patients do want to see the inside of their cervix and uterine cavity, and doing so allays some of the anxiety associated with the procedure. It is also helpful for nursing assistants to simultaneously view the procedure so that they know when more pressure or flow of distention media is necessary. The image of the uterine cavity through the hysteroscope is just a few millimeters in diameter. With video, the image can be enlarged to a size to which the surgeon is more accustomed. Without video documentation, the surgeon must diagram the hysteroscopic findings in the patient record. With the use of a video mavigraph, an instant photo is obtained and can be stapled in the record for permanent documentation.

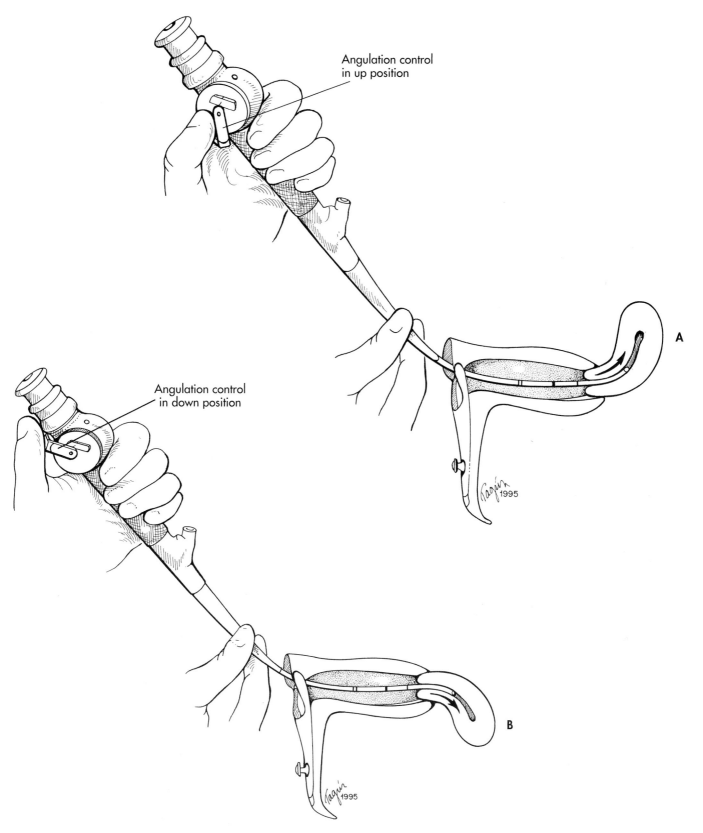

Angulation control
in up position

Angulation control
in down position

A

B

Fig. 3-6. Insertion of a flexible hysteroscope into a uterus. **A,** The flexible hysteroscope is guided into the anteflexed endometrial cavity by deflection of the distal end using the thumb manipulator. **B,** The flexible hysteroscope is guided into the retroflexed endometrial cavity also by deflection of its distal end using the thumb manipulator.

The significant disadvantage of a video setup is cost. At the very least it will add $3000 to $5000 to the hysteroscopic system. Depending on the equipment purchased, the cost could exceed $20,000. A video system consists of a camera and coupler, video monitor, and cart. Video documentation can include a video recorder and/or a video mavigraph

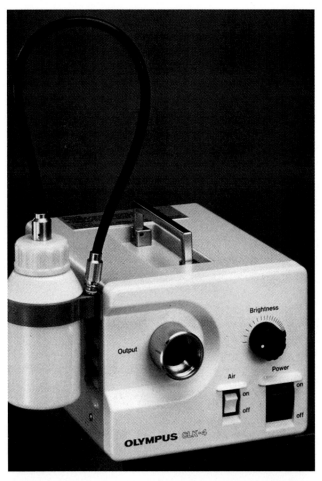

Fig. 3-7. 150 W halogen light source. (Courtesy Olympus America, Inc, Medical Instruments Division, Lake Success, NY.)

and/or a slidemaker. As mentioned, the mavigraph is very useful for documentation in the patient record. A video recorder and slidemaker are necessary only for teaching purposes.

Video camera. One chip, two chip, three chip, digital or analog, 2 dimension, or 3 dimension: What does it mean and which camera is needed for office hysteroscopy? Older cameras consisted of television tubes to electronically process an image and send the image to a monitor. Although the image was of good quality, the camera itself was bulky. Newer video cameras contain a charge-couple device (CCD) chip composed of approximately 400,000 light-sensitive elements.[3] When light strikes the silicon device, electrical resistance of the silicon decreases, thereby generating current carriers. The photosensitive silicon elements transfer information as packets of electrical charge, or pixels, which are then amplified. The number of pixels determines the number of lines of resolution (420 to 480) of the camera, which, in turn, determines the sharpness of the picture. While it is true that if one chip is good then three chips must be better, the additional expense of a three-chip camera does not justify its use in office hysteroscopy. Currently, we are using office hysteroscopy to identify macroscopic lesions, and the single-chip cameras provide more than enough clarity to do this.

CCD video cameras are lightweight and connected with a cable to the camera control unit (CCU). They can be immersed in disinfecting solutions but in general do not need to be sterile for diagnostic office hysteroscopy. The CCD video camera contains an iris that will adjust to the light intensity to compensate for light reflection. The CCU will adjust the light from the light source as well as the color and white balance.

At present no true digital CCDs are available commercially. All signals that leave each individual pixel on the CCD are analog. A digital camera uses digital signal processing (DSP) (Fig. 3-9). DSP takes the video information that is delivered from the CCD chip and digitizes it. Through digitization, background noise is reduced, brightness is increased, and the sharpness and edge

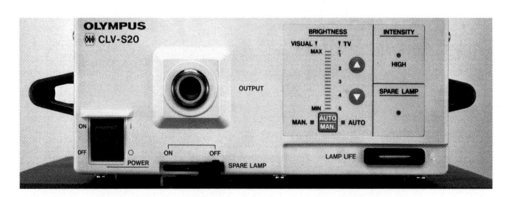

Fig. 3-8. 300 W xenon light source (Courtesy Olympus America, Inc, Medical Instruments Division, Lake Success, NY.)

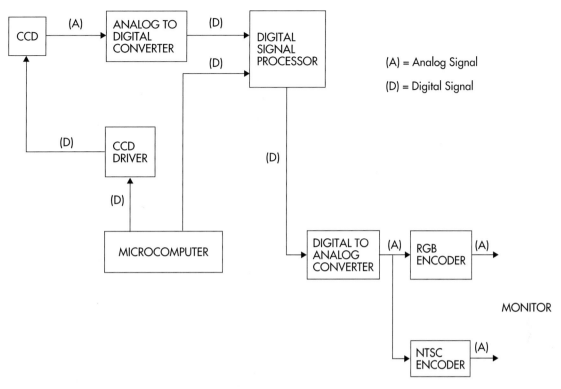

Fig. 3-9. Digital camera system with digital signal processing (DSP). DSP takes the video information and digitizes it, providing increased brightness and sharpness to the image. This DSP is specific
to Olympus America. Other types of digital enhancement are used by other companies.

enhancement of the video image is improved. The digitization of the video image is analogous to the digitization
of an audio compact disk. When music is digitized, the
processing circuitry removes a significant amount of
unwanted noise. The digital information is then converted
back to the analog equivalent before being displayed
on the video monitor. With digital signal processing a
minimum of 3 lux are needed for proper visualization. Without digital processing a minimum of 15 lux are necessary.

When using the flexible hysteroscope, the image will have
a honeycomb appearance unless a moiré-reducing filter is
placed on the camera. With the use of this filter, the image has
a smooth appearance similar to that of a rigid hysteroscope.

Camera coupler. The camera is mounted onto the eyepiece of the hysteroscope by a coupler. The coupler may be
direct, whereby the image can only be seen on a video monitor, or it may be coupled with a beam splitter. The beam
splitter allows one to view the image directly through the
hysteroscope or on the video monitor. The beam splitter,
however, will cause a 30% reduction of light from the light
source to the uterine cavity (Fig. 3-10, *A*). The camera coupler is furnished with a focusing ring and occasionally a
zoom ring for magnification (Fig. 3-10, *B*). Camera couplers
are available with rotating heads, which allow the surgeon
to rotate the hysteroscope while keeping the camera in
its proper orientation. Electronic video endoscopes contain

the video chip within the distal end of the hysteroscope
(Fig. 3-10, *C*). These instruments are currently being used in
gastroenterology and will become available in future generations of flexible hysteroscopes.

Color monitors

Depending on the size of the examination room and the
video cart being used, the color monitor should be between
9 and 20 inches in diameter. The smaller screens will improve the sharpness of the image; however, the larger screen
is essential if the monitor is placed in a position for patient,
assistant, and operator viewing. Assuming the same illumination, a 40% larger image will appear half as bright on the
television screen.

The low-end monitors will have between 350 and 450
lines of resolution with the standard BNC composite connections. This resolution is sufficient when using the smaller
9-inch monitors. When using a monitor equal to or larger
than 13 inches, a high resolution (600 to 750 lines of resolution) should be employed. These monitors will come with
BNC composite terminals as well as RGB (red, green, blue)
connectors to allow fine tuning of the color image. In addition, the higher-grade monitors offer automatic white balance, an overscan mode to increase magnification of the image up to 117%, and single or dual VHS terminals for
connection of additional monitors if desired.

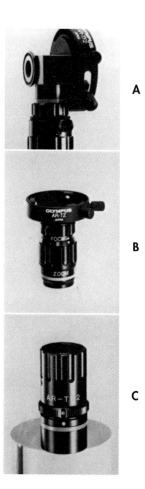

Fig. 3-10. **A,** Beam splitter camera coupler. The beam splitter allows one to view the image directly through the hysteroscope or on the video monitor. This beam splitter has a rotating head, which will keep the camera properly oriented. **B,** Direct camera coupler. This coupler is furnished with a focusing ring and a zoom ring for magnification. **C,** Internal video camera. An internal video chip is used in place of an eyepiece on the hysteroscope. With this system the image can be seen only through the video camera. (Courtesy Olympus America, Inc, Medical Instruments Division, Lake Success, NY.)

Video printers

Video printers convert video images to hard-copy prints. Today's printers use thermal color printing in which a heated printhead is used to melt dots of colored wax or plastic onto paper. With an RGB full-frame memory, the input video signal is digitally processed in 8 bits (256 gradations) and more than 16 million colors per dot. This produces more than 500 TV lines of resolution in an image of 708 (H) $\times$ 448 (V) dots (Fig. 3-11). The images are produced in approximately 20 to 80 seconds, depending on the model printer used. Most printers have a multiprint mode in which multiple images can be captured on one print. This capability is useful in office hysteroscopy when one wants to document the visualization of both tubal ostia as well as any intrauterine pathology.

Video recorders and slidemakers

Video recorders and slidemakers are used chiefly for teaching. Video recorders are available in three-quarter inch or half-inch formats. The three-quarter inch format provides a better quality with less distortion than the half-inch tape. However, the standard home VCR is half-inch format, and unless one is producing films for large audiences with significant editing necessary, the half-inch format is sufficient and less expensive.

Medical quality half-inch video recorders are available that have features not found on home recorders. For example, the Sony SVO-1410 model has not only high quality (HQ) and 4-head design (just as the home models), but also features such as a quick-response mechanism to provide rapid access to video images, digital auto tracking, and auto repeat function to play back a particular hysteroscopic image automatically.

Video slide-making systems are available that will produce high-resolution 35-mm slides from any standard video signal (Fig. 3-12). The printers are designed to work in unison with video printers. The color resolution is 8 bits per primary color (256 gradations), and the video signal is in the RGB format from the video printer. The Sony SlidemakerMD comes with a foot pedal that allows the operator to select either a slide image or a mavigraph image to be recorded. The slides take about 20 seconds to be captured on standard 100 ISO, 35-mm film.

Hysteroscopy cart

Any makeshift cart will be sufficient as long as it provides enough stability for the equipment. However, if expensive video equipment is being used, it would behoove the surgeon to purchase a video cart that is both stable and mobile, and provides electrical plugs with surge protection for all the equipment.

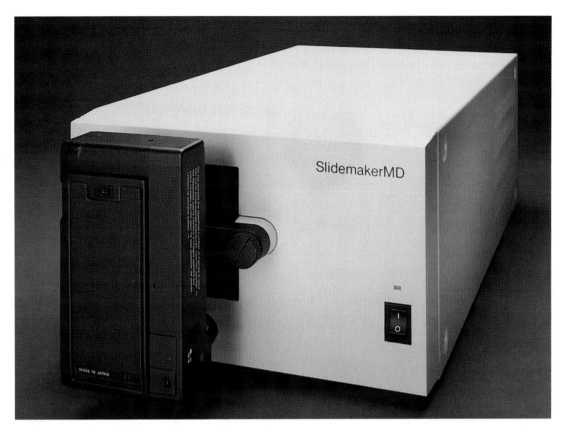

Fig. 3-11. Video slidemaker. This unit produces high-resolution 35-mm slides from a video signal. (Courtesy Olympus America, Inc, Medical Instruments Division, Lake Success, NY.)

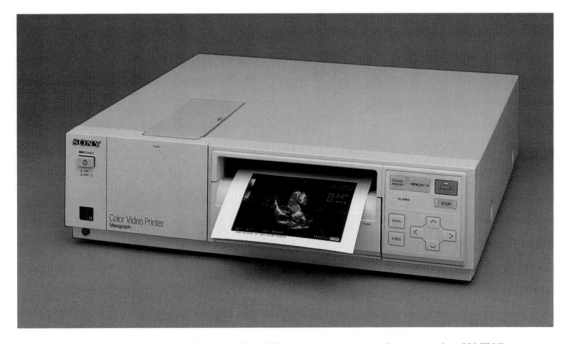

Fig. 3-12. Video mavigraph. This Sony UP-2200 color video printer produces more than 500 TV lines of resolution. (Courtesy Olympus America, Inc, Medical Instruments Division, Lake Success, NY.)

The basic office hysteroscopy cart is a small footprint cart with a soaking basin for flexible hysteroscope disinfection, a top shelf, and two additional shelves. A 9- to 20-inch monitor can be placed on top of the cart. Also available is a video cart with a swing arm for a 9- to 13-inch monitor. This cart is slightly larger than the standard cart and has four shelves. The swing arm allows the monitor to be placed directly in front of the surgeon's face just over the patient's abdomen (Fig. 3-13). In this manner the surgeon can face forward while performing the hysteroscopy. Unless a second monitor is used, however, the patient and assistant will not be able to view the procedure.

Costs

Because costs are constantly changing, it is impossible to provide updated figures from every manufacturer. Costs will vary from year to year as new technology becomes available. In addition, costs will depend on whether equipment is purchased separately or in a package. Below is a sample of

office hysteroscopy equipment available from Olympus with the prices as of April 1994.

Obviously many combinations of equipment are available for office hysteroscopy. The appropriate system for

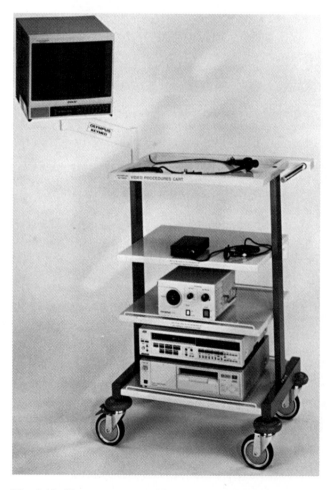

Fig. 3-13. Hysteroscopy cart. Video cart with four shelves and a swing arm that will accommodate monitors from 9 to 13 inches. (Courtesy Olympus America, Inc, Medical Instruments Division, Lake Success, NY.)

Sample of office hysteroscopy equipment and costs

Hysteroscopes

Rigid 3-mm hysteroscope with 4-mm sheath	$3650
Flexible 3.6-mm HYF-P hysteroscope	$6300
Continuous-flow 5.5-mm rigid hysteroscope with semi-rigid instruments	$7700
Flexible 4.9-mm HYF-1T hysteroscope	$6900

Light sources

150 W halogen	$780
175 W xenon	$4680
300 W xenon	$8630

Carbon dioxide insufflator	$2030

Cameras

Nondigital, nonimmersible camera, with coupler	$3700
Digital camera with moiré filter	$9500
Three-chip camera	$19,000

Color monitors

9-inch standard monitor	$435
13-inch high-resolution monitor	$1225
20-inch high-resolution monitor	$2112

Video printers

Sony UP-2200	$1680
Sony UP-3000	$3360

Video recorders

SVO-1410 standard half-inch format	$500
SVO-9500 half-inch hospital grade	$2295

Video slidemaker

SlidemakerMD	$2795

Video carts

Standard cart	$1165
Video cart with articulating arm	$2400

Packages available

3.6-mm flexible scope plus 150 W light source	$6920
Above plus cart	$7985
Above with least expensive video system (including 175 W light source)	$15,430
Above with digital camera	$18,030
Above with high-resolution monitor, and hard-copy video printer (UP-2200)	$23,677
Above with UP-3000 video printer, VCR recorder, SlidemakerMD	$27,126

each physician will depend on personal preference, patient volume, and reimbursement. At Massachusetts General Hospital, the CPT code for diagnostic office hysteroscopy is 56350, with a surgical fee of $450 per procedure.

REFERENCES

1. Baggish MS: Initiating a hysteroscopic programme. In Sutton and Diamond MP, Eds: *Endoscopic surgery for gynaecologists,* Philadelphia, 1993, W.B. Saunders Co.

2. Buyalos RP: Principles of endoscopic optics and lighting. In Azziz R, Murphy AA, Eds: *Practical manual of operative laparoscopy and hysteroscopy,* New York, 1992, Springer-Verlag.

3. Azziz R: Photo and video documentation in endoscopic surgery. In Azziz R, Murphy AA, Eds: *Practical manual of operative laparoscopy and hysteroscopy,* New York, 1992, Springer-Verlag.

Chapter 4

FLEXIBLE HYSTEROSCOPY INSTRUMENTATION

René Marty
Patricia Mussuto

Uterine endoscopy is one of the oldest techniques employed in gynecology. For a long time, however, its evolution was hindered by use of hysteroscopes that were not adapted to the dimensions and tissue consistency of the uterus.

Over the past 100 years we have experienced the development of a hysteroscopic technique (deemed conventional) that relies on the use of rigid optics. However, examination is limited in that there are intracavitary obstacles that cannot be bypassed using rigid optics without the risk of uterine trauma.

It was in this context that in 1968 Mohri[1] decided to use a flexible endoscope within the uterus to view as closely as possible the fetus of a post-term woman.

The ability to deflect the optical fiber equipment has enabled the use of flexible hysteroscopy to expand rapidly. In addition to its numerous diagnostic and endoscopic surgical indications, the flexible hysteroscope can aid in assisted reproductive technologies, and it seems to have revolutionary prospects in infertility falloposcopy.

Flexible hysteroscopy can be used no matter what the intracavitary dimensions may be. In addition, patients' ages do not constitute a major obstacle.

HISTORY OF FLEXIBLE HYSTEROSCOPY

In the 1960s, at the Yokusuka Clinic in Japan, gynecologists Takaaki and Chi Mohri[1] were working on a method for antenatal diagnosis of fetal malformations. They were the first gynecologists in the world to present a film on fetal movements. The film was instrumental in the arrival of the first hysterofiberscope in endoscopy on Nov. 8, 1963.

This endoscope, which was entirely flexible, stemmed from a series of technologic steps and medical research. In 1870 the physicist Tyndall discovered that a beam of light

could be transmitted from glass fibers. In 1928 Baird resumed the study and developed the transmission of pictures by regrouping glass and quartz fibers. Hansell demonstrated the power of resistance of this equipment in 1930, and Van Heel developed a method to channel and avoid the anarchic diffusion of information by covering the beams with a material containing a low refraction index. In 1954 Hopkins improved the manufacturing of these fibers and increased their market production. At the same time, he sorted out the theory of light beams and image transmission.

The complete flexibility of these fibers was recognized as early as 1870. This quality became essential in the investigation of hollow organs. In 1954 Hirschowitz[2] created the first gastroduodenal fiberscope, which enabled him to reach bulbar lesions. An esophagoscope was the second flexible fiberscope created on the advice of physicians Philips and Presti.

It was not until 10 years after the creation of the gastroduodenoscope that this technique was used in gynecology and obstetrics. As mentioned, Mohri recorded fetal images in pregnancies doomed to therapeutic abortion or in post-term pregnancies. The gestational age of these pregnancies ranged from 5 to 10 months.

Evolution from the first hysterofiberscope

The distal part of Mohri's first endoscope[1] employed a 6 V vacuum light bulb that was responsible for a foreoblique diffusion of light with a field angle of 60°. The distal objective consisted of a prism and a convergent lens that focused the image on the distal part of the beam.[1]

The body of the endoscope, which contained the entire image transmission and light network, was completely flexible and protected by a stainless steel spiral that was also covered by a plastic-coated, smooth sheath. The proximal objective created a 10-fold magnification. Water was used for insufflation, and the connection was done by an insufflation bulb. A 12 V transformer provided electrical power. The total length of the endoscope was 65 cm, with an outer diameter of 12 mm.

The image was transmitted via a consistent beam in which the fibers were oriented the same way from the proximal to the distal part. Each 15-μm fiber was responsible for an infinitesimal part of the image. Hirschowitz's gastroduodenoscope enclosed 150,000 glass fibers with a total optical diameter of 6 mm. The hysterofiberscope held only 40,000 fibers three decades later.[2] It had a diameter of 4 mm and better resolution, and could transmit information two and a half times faster. The hysterofiberscope also featured the optical isolation of each fiber bundle through a sheath, which decreased loss of information within it.

Within 7 years, the Japanese school had perfected this hysterofiberscope. The lighting system, which used a lamp under vacuum, was replaced by a system that kept the light source out of the uterus. This modification allowed a reduction in the diameter of the endoscope to 7 mm from 12 mm, thus making the procedure easier to use with nulliparous women.

The flexible method remained unknown in Europe and the United States until 1974. At that time, the Japanese reported on the use of the flexible device and its advantages at the World Congress in Rio de Janeiro.

Although rigid hysteroscopy was being widely used between 1975 and 1985, a growing number of gynecologists began to use the flexible device. Studies were published as early as 1988 in Europe[3,4] and the United States. Over the past 5 years, flexible hysteroscopy has expanded again, with France playing a key role.[4,5]

UNDERSTANDING THE ANATOMY BEFORE HYSTEROSCOPY

It is important to understand cervical and uterine anatomy before performing office hysteroscopy. It is because of these dimensions, as well as the angulation between the cervix and the uterus, that the flexible hysteroscope was developed.[5]

The uterus takes the shape of a truncated cone tightened at the middle—the isthmus. This area separates the corpus from the cervix.

In the nulliparous woman, the uterus is, on average, 7.5 cm long (i.e., about 3.5 cm for the corpus and 2.5 cm for the cervix, with the isthmus being 1.5 cm long). The corpus is 4 cm wide, and the cervix is 2.5 cm wide. In multiparous women, the length of the uterus ranges from 7 to 10 cm (5 to 5.5 cm for the corpus and 2 to 2.5 cm for the cervix). The width at the base of the corpus reaches 5 cm and does not exceed 3 cm at the middle of the uterus (Table 4-1). In menopausal women these figures can become greatly reduced, varying according to the time elapsed between the beginning of menopause and the examination.

The consistency and length of the cervix vary according to the reproduction period of the woman. In the nulliparous

Table 4-1. Average outer uterine dimensions

	Nulliparous		Multiparous	
	Length	*Width*	*Length*	*Width*
Corpus	3.5 cm	4 cm	5.5 cm	5 cm
Isthmus	1.5 cm		1.5 cm	
Cervix	2.5 cm	2 cm	2.5 cm	3 cm
TOTAL	7.5 cm		7-10 cm	

woman, the outer orifice of the cervix is circular with a diameter of 5 to 6 mm. In the primiparous woman, the top of the muzzle flattens out and the outer orifice lengthens transversely. In the multiparous woman, the intravaginal side of the cervix lengthens, and the outer orifice can reach a diameter of 15 mm. In the menopausal woman, the orifice will often fibrose and lose its elasticity, which can lead to sclerotic obliteration.

The uterine cavity corresponds to the virtual space that is to be cautiously dilated to allow a panoramic view of the corpus. It is 25 to 35 mm long, while the isthmus is 5 mm long and the cervix 25 mm long. The intracavitary dimensions of the two segments are stable despite a history of gestation.

CHARACTERISTICS OF FLEXIBLE HYSTEROFIBERSCOPES

The *flexible hysteroscope* is a generic term for two types of hysterofiberscopes: diagnostic and therapeutic.

Their fundamental features are flexibility, airtightness, and optical fibers. Their differences lie in the dimensions and the choice of materials used by the manufacturers: Olympus,[6] Fuji, Storz, Leisegang, Machida, and Wolf. The flexible hysteroscope comprises four parts: (1) a case, (2) a sheath that links it to the (3) bendable extremity, and (4) a connection link to the light source (Fig. 4-1).

The case (proximal extremity)

The case is lightweight and easily held by the operator. A remote control lever for the bendable segment is present on one side of the proximal extremity. The case holds the proximal optical system, which comprises the ocular and dioptrical adjustment ring; the entrance orifice of the operative canal, which, depending on the devices, is or is not equipped with an airtight valve; and the departure of the fiberscope sheath, which is located at the distal part of the case.

The main sheath

In most of the devices currently available, the main sheath is completely flexible. An exception is the Fuji endoscope, which will be discussed later. This pliable segment is relatively resistant to torsion. The movements that are applied to it are directly transmitted to the distal segment. The main sheath contains the conducting beam of the image, the lighting beams, and the operative canal (whose dimensions are detailed in the comparative tables on page 34). The sheath is

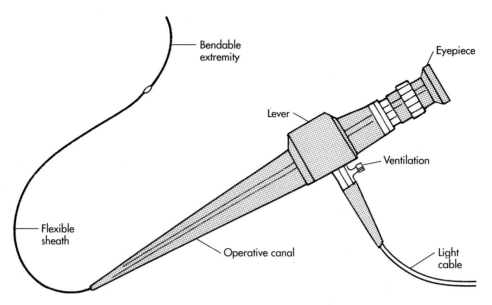

Fig. 4-1. Flexible diagnostic hysteroscope.

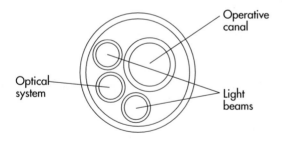

Fig. 4-2. Nontraumatic distal extremity of the hysteroscope.

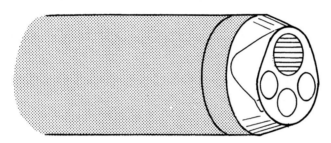

Fig. 4-3. Transverse section of the distal extremity.

perfectly airtight and is composed of a steel mesh whose pliability depends on the length and thickness of the material.

The distal extremity

The distal extremity of the flexible fiberscope enables the operator to get an axial view of the uterine cavity. The bendable extremity can be manipulated in at least four directions within the uterine cavity (i.e., up, down, left, and right). The ultimate direction of the distal extremity is determined by

the movements on the sheath combined with the use of the thumb lever. The distal tip of the endoscope comprises a nontraumatic rim. On a transverse section, the objective is located under the operative canal and is surrounded by lighting beams (Fig. 4-2).

The light connection

The light connection shelters all the optical components in a sheath identical to that of the fiberscope. This part, which most often cannot be dissociated from the case, ends with a plug that is usually specific to the light source. Adapters connect the endoscope to different types of light sources, but the luminosity decreases by at least 20% with each intermediary.

The operative canal. The diameter of the operative canal ranges from 1 mm for the diagnostic hysteroscope to 2.2 mm for the therapeutic hysteroscope. The canal is used by both the distention medium and supplementary instruments such as biopsy forceps and laser fibers. Thus it appears that the most effective device should have the smallest possible O.D., with an operative canal at least 1.2 mm wide (the thinnest diameter for an instrument being 1 mm) (Fig. 4-3).

Microstructure of the optical system. The optical fibers are organized in two categories of bundles. The bundle that carries the image to the eyepiece is coherent and is responsible for the transmission of the image to the eyepiece; the second bundle is noncoherent and conveys the light into the uterine cavity (Fig. 4-4). There are usually two noncoherent bundles per hysteroscope.[6,7]

To transmit an image, a fiber beam must be coupled at both extremities with a system of convergent lenses. The image appears on the distal section through a lens system that constitutes the objective and whose focal distance determines the field angle. The image is conveyed to the beam's

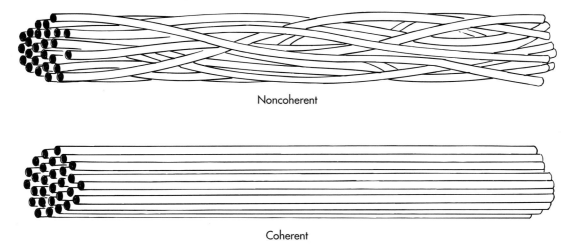

Noncoherent

Coherent

Fig. 4-4. Optical fiber beams. (*Top,* noncoherent; *bottom,* coherent).

proximal section, where another system of lenses makes up the ocular and ensures a 10- to 20-fold enlargement. This ocular can be adjusted to the eyesight of the endoscopist. The information is sent by a coherent beam, which is composed of glass fibers that are similarly arranged from one extremity to the other. The image is then split up into as many points as there are optical fibers. The diameter of the fibers ranges from 6 to 13 µm.

The number and thinness of the optical fibers do not appear to be a criterion of quality (Fig. 4-5). The thinner and longer the fibers are, the more information that is lost. Gaps that occur when the fibers are assembled can distort the image. When the refraction index of this component is low, the loss of information is reduced. The obvious advantage of these flexible fibers compared with the conventional rigid optical system is the ability to convey the image no matter what the degree of curvature.

The noncoherent beams are assemblages of optical fibers that are haphazardly arranged. They are coupled with another lens system and extended without interruption from the external light source to the distal extremity of the fiberscope, therefore requiring a good lighting power.

Summary of flexible endoscopic components

The various endoscopic features of a flexible hysteroscope comprise the direct lighting, the field angle, the depth of the field, the bending degree, the inner diameter, the usable length, the total length, the operative canal, and the possible connections of the hysteroscope.

These data are grouped in comparative charts by diagnostic or operative category (Tables 4-2 and 4-3).

COMPLEMENTARY TOOLS

Biopsy forceps

Operators agree that biopsy forceps are vital instruments for hysteroscopy. Being able to sample an endometrial lesion under direct visualization is an integral function

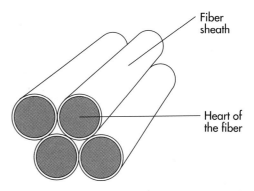

Fiber sheath

Heart of the fiber

Fig. 4-5. Structure of optical fibers.

of office hysteroscopy. This capability should eventually replace the "blind" D&C for ruling out endometrial pathology. The three leading manufacturers of biopsy instruments—Olympus, Cook, and Fuji—have provided several types of nozzles that enable the surgeon to choose forceps appropriate to the topography of the lesion to be removed.

Whatever the extremity of the forceps may be, their diameter must be smaller than that of the operative canal, which is 1 to 2.2 mm.

The Fujinon HYSF or HYSR is not compatible with a biopsy during eye-controlled hysteroscopy. Its operative canal is 1 mm in diameter, which does not allow the simultaneous passage of the forceps and the liquid medium unlike the Fujinon HYSFP, with its 1.2 mm canal. With diagnostic flexible hysteroscopy, the 3 French standard forceps offers a tissue volume of 0.86 mm.[3] The 5 French "standard cup" and "elongated cup" forceps measure 2.25 mm^3 and 4.85 mm^3 respectively and are used during a surgical endoscopy.

From the three manufacturers mentioned above, four types of biopsy forceps are at the disposal of the endoscopist (Fig. 4-6):

The "rat tooth" is a standard forceps in the shape of a full hollow cup (Fuji) or oblong (Cook). It is indicated for a frontal approach sampling.

Table 4-2. Comparison of flexible diagnostic hysteroscopes

Components	Olympus HYF-P	Fujinon* HYSF/HYSR	Machida* FS HYS	Storz	Leisegang LMFLEY	Circon Series AUR-FH
Lighting	Direct	Direct	Direct	Direct	Direct	
Field angle	90°	90°	80°	100°	95°	85°
Depth of field	1-50 mm	1-50 mm	3-50 mm	1-50 mm	1-50 mm	
Bendable section	100°–top 100°–bottom	100°–top 90°–bottom	100°–top 90°–bottom	180°–top 100°–bottom	100°–top 100°–bottom	160°
Outer diameter	3.6 mm	3.7 mm	3.6 mm	3.5 mm	3.6 mm	3.25 mm
Usable length	160 mm	210 mm	215 mm	340 mm	250 mm	200 mm
Total length	540 mm	580 mm	600 mm		525 mm	
Diameter of operative canal	1.2 mm	1 mm	1 mm	1.2 mm	1.2 mm	1.2 mm

*Fujinon and Machida are a semiflexible intermediate generation.

The sheath of the diagnostic semiflexible fiberscope comprises three parts: (1) the flexible proximal segment, which allows the operator to have a comfortable posture and avoids contortion; (2) the rigid intermediate segment, which eases the transition from rigid to completely flexible endoscope; and (3) the flexible distal segment, which is common to all other bendable extremities and endows the endoscope with all the qualities of flexible devices.

Table 4-3. Comparison of flexible therapeutic hysteroscopes

	OLYMPUS HYF Type 1T	FUJINON HYS-FI'/I-IYS-RT
Lighting	Direct	Direct
Field angle	120° retrograde view	90° retrograde view
Depth of field	2-50 mm	1-50 mm
Outer diameter	4.9 mm	4.8 mm
Diameter of distal extremity	4.5 mm	4.8 mm
Bendable section*	120° top 120° bottom	100° top 90° bottom
Total length	590 mm	590 mm
Useful length	290 mm	205 mm
Diameter of operative canal	2.2 mm	2 mm
Axis rotation†		140°
Connection angle on semiflexible part‡		45°

*The evolution of endoscopes shows that the bending angle does not need to be above 100°. This point differs from gastroduodenoscopes, which have difficulty controlling the cardia because of their curves.

†The semiflexible therapeutic Fujinon has an additional characteristic compared with the diagnostic endoscope. A ring is inserted in the initial part of the segment, giving it a 140° axle rotation. This feature increases the comfort of the operator.

‡The Fujinon hysteroscope with two segments at sheath level: one rigid and proximal, the other flexible and distal.

The "alligator forceps," available in 3 and 5 French diameters, is used for an oblique preemption when the frontal take becomes delicate.

The "rat tooth with needle," in the shape of a hollow cup that contains a thin needle between its two jaws, was designed to set and carry samples of mobile, intracavitary elements such as small polyps or pedicled fibromas.

The "mouse tooth forceps," the last type manufactured by Cook, has a 3 French diameter, and its cup shape is completed by two opposed hooks at its distal part. It is indicated when obtaining a tissue sample for biopsy from an atrophic endometrium in the menopausal woman or when obtaining a specimen of submucous myomata for biopsy.

The German manufacturer Storz has a range of additional instruments similar to those just mentioned (i.e., standard biopsy forceps and forceps with jaws to grasp the sample more firmly). The latter are available with a 3 French diameter or a 7 French diameter (not usable in the flexible endoscope).

Polyp snares

For the removal of small polyps with a narrow pedicle, we have at our disposal the Olympus FG 39 SX, shaped like a lasso, and the Fuji basket (Fig. 4-7). Polypectomy with either of these devices provides for both anatomic-pathologic diagnosis and therapeutic treatment. When intrauterine devices are embedded into the myometrium or when there remains only one part of a polyp that is difficult to remove by eye control, tools such as the Olympus FG 40 ST or the Fuji forceps with three teeth can be very useful.

Monopolar electrodes

Monopolar electrodes can be used through a 2-mm operative canal and are indicated for electrocoagulation. They cannot be used in an electrolyte-containing liquid medium such as saline or lactated Ringer's. Ideally, polypectomies and pedicle coagulation should be performed using the laser. However, because current lasers are expensive and difficult to obtain, monopolar electrodes may be employed instead, using CO_2 to distend the uterus.

DESCRIPTION OF THE ENDOSCOPIC ACT

Preparing for the examination

One of the principles of flexible hysteroscopy is to personalize the examination. Because the instruments used in fiberhysteroscopy are small, anesthesia is used only in very specific cases, such as with some postmenopausal

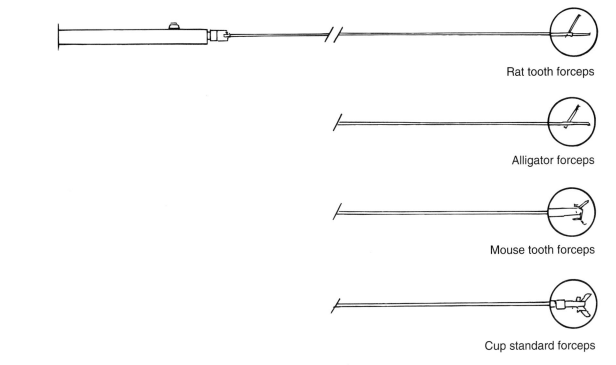

Figure 4-6. Cook biopsy forceps.

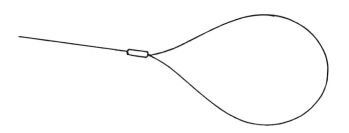

Fig. 4-7. Olympus lasso for polypectomy.

women or patients who already have had cervical surgery; the cervix of these patients is fibrotic and narrow. This idea relies on detailed patient education describing the procedure (See Chapter 5). In most cases, because the hysteroscope's eyepiece is equipped with a camera, patients will be able to observe the hysteroscopic procedure on the television screen.[3]

The hysteroscopic examination must be preceded by an essential first step: the gynecologic consultation and examination. The goal is to determine the dimensions of the uterus and the cervical orifice by pelvic examinations and hysterometry.

The results of these examinations are then compared with the age of the patient. If there is the slightest doubt as to vaginal or adnexal infection, the examination will be postponed until after bacteriologic samples have been obtained and appropriate antibiotic treatment given. If the tests are negative, the physician will prescribe local antiseptics (one vaginal pellet to be taken every night for 6 days until the day before the examination). The patient's gynecologic and general personal history is obtained to assist in understanding the presence of

lesions noted during hysteroscopy. For example, in patients with a prior myomectomy, we will look for a deformation of the uterine cavity. In patients with a prior cesarean section we will look for an anterior low uterine scar and with a history of an induced abortion or D&C following a delivery, the presence of synechiae.

During the gynecologic consultation, the question of whether to use local or no anesthesia is raised. We rarely choose local anesthesia, reserving it only for patients with a stenotic cervix who require dilatation of the internal cervical os. Dilatation of the external cervical os can be done painlessly. One must keep in mind that office hysteroscopy is easier and quicker when the patient is relaxed, therefore, most diagnostic hysteroscopies, as well as those undertaken to obtain biopsy samples, are performed without anesthesia. Dialogue between the physician, the assistant, and the patient acts as verbal anesthesia.

The day of the examination

The patient must arrive 30 minutes before the examination and insert an antispasmodic suppository. She is informed about the gynecologic position to take after she has emptied her bladder and is then interviewed to ascertain one final time the date of her last menstrual period because the examination must be performed during the first part of her cycle and preferably before the twelfth day. This interview takes into account the presence or absence of spotting or menometrorrhagia during the past 48 hours, ongoing or recently interrupted hormonal treatment, and the presence of an IUD. Although this information was obtained during the gynecologic consultation, it should be solicited again to record on the anatomic-pathology sheet because it can ease interpretation of the report.

The equipment is then presented: camera, television screen, and hysteroscope, while the tray is being brought forward. On the sterile tray are the Pozzi forceps, long atraumatic forceps, sterile compresses, a disposal receptacle for the povidone-iodine (Betadine) solution, and a container to recover the biopsy fragments before placing them in the fixative. A flexible hysterometer is also put on the tray and, as a precaution, a range of flexible dilators in case the inner cervical orifice would have to be gently dilated to avoid any tearing from an ill-prepared pathway.

The operator takes a comfortable sitting position directly in front of the patient and controls the endoscopic act by referring to the television screen. Flexible hysteroscopy, unlike rigid hysteroscopy, requires no operator contortion. The light connections and the hook-up of the liquid medium to the hysteroscope are done very quickly.

The adjustment of the camera (i.e., focus and white balance) is preceded by one last adjustment of the optics on the hysteroscope so that the endoscopist will have the clearest possible view.

The flexible hysteroscope is inserted through the external cervical os, with the device in the straight position. Unlike rigid hysteroscopy, there is usually no need to use a tenaculum to stabilize the cervix or straighten the canal. When the distal extremity is within the cervical canal, the image on the television monitor will be all white to pink. At this time, the liquid medium should be instilled under pressure and the hysteroscope withdrawn slightly until the internal cervical os is clearly visualized.

When instilling the distention medium, the operator will dilate the cervical canal slightly to allow slow advancement of the tip of the hysteroscope through the internal os into the uterine cavity using a no-touch technique. This means that the hysteroscope should be advanced when the canal is in the middle of the television screen. If the canal is off center, the scope will angle into the cervical or endometrial wall. If the tip of the hysteroscope goes up against the cervical wall while the scope is being advanced, the entire screen will appear white. The scope should again be withdrawn slowly until the cervical canal or endometrial cavity is clearly seen. The angles of the cervical canal and lower uterine segment can be maneuvered painlessly by guiding the distal extremity with the thumb manipulator (Fig. 4-8).

The progression of the device must be slow so the various intracavitary landmarks can be located: the cervical canal, the internal cervical ostia, the isthmus of the uterus, and the tubal orifices. If all of these landmarks are not visualized, the examination should not be considered complete. Once all of the landmarks have been identified, the hysteroscope is withdrawn to the level of the lower uterine cavity to allow a general panoramic view of the uterine cavity. One can notice its normal, deformed, or cylindric aspects, as well as its obstruction by an intracavitary malformation. One can

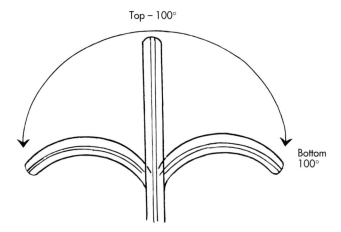

Fig. 4-8. Bendable extremity of pliable hysteroscope.

also note any intracavitary lesions such as myomata or polyps.

If the panoramic view of the cavity does not reveal any particular abnormality, a detailed examination of the cavity should be undertaken. The anterior and posterior walls of the uterus can be examined by pushing the thumb manipulator up or down. If the operator then rotates the case of the hysteroscope by 90°, the manipulator can be displaced to visualize the lateral walls as well (Fig. 4-9). Similar maneuvers can be done with the tip of the scope near the tubal orifices to obtain a detailed examination. The depth of the tubal ostium, its possible funnel shape, and the contractions that may be visible from the tubal orifice should be noted.

Each wall of the uterus is thoroughly examined. The examination should first be done from a distance to detect any interstitial or pedicled formation, and then close up to clearly visualize the vascular pattern or an adenomyosis.

Apart from visual analysis of the thickness of the endometrium, whether it has a thin and fibrous or thick and fluffy coating can be determined by using repeated pressure to place the endoscope in physical contact at different levels of the endometrium.

In the presence of an intracavitary malformation, the first aim is to determine its level of implantation and assess its size and surface area. These data will influence the subsequent therapeutic choice. For example, if there is a submucous myoma that is 50% intramural and 50% submucous, the patient should be informed that a hysteroscopic resection may require a two-stage procedure. No part of these lesions, including what might be hidden behind, should remain unexplored.

The endoscope is withdrawn from the intrauterine cavity only after pathologic or cytologic samples have been taken under direct visualization. As a rule, biopsies are never performed randomly. The biopsy forceps can easily be placed opposite the endometrial area or intracavitary element if the lesion is sessile or mobile. The appraisal of the thickness of the endometrium, as well as altered topography caused by a

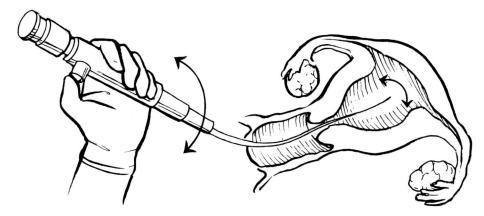

Fig. 4-9. Diagnostic hysteroscopy endoscope.

lesion, will determine the appropriate choice of forceps.

Several samples can be taken without inducing bleeding, which would hamper visibility. Some fragments are placed in a receptacle containing salt solution to measure their size before placing them in the fixative.

The flexible hysteroscope is withdrawn as slowly as it was inserted to schematize all lesions detected from a frontal or a sagittal section for inclusion in the patient's record.

This identification sheet both summarizes the examination and records the topography of any lesions and the context in which the examination was carried out. It should also include the duration of the procedure, the volume of the distention solution employed, the type of hysteroscope used, the number of biopsy samples obtained, and the therapy considered.

The duration of the diagnostic examination is about 5 to 10 minutes. The actual time necessary to visualize the entire uterine cavity rarely exceeds 45 to 60 seconds. When various biopsy forceps are used, the duration of the procedure rarely exceeds 15 minutes.

In this context and without anesthesia, the patient lies or sits to recover for about 5 minutes and then goes back to a normal activity.

REFERENCES

1. Mohri C, Yamadori F: Problem of observing the human ovum descending in the fallopian tube by a tubaloscope. In Morhi T, and Mohri C, Eds: *Our 25 years experience with endoscope,* Japan, 1968.
2. Hirschowitz: Endoscopic examination of the stomach and duodenal cup with the fiberscope, *Lancet,* 1:1074-1078, 1954.
3. Marty R: A propos de la fibro-hysteroscopie souple diagnostic et operatoire, *Contracept Fertil Sex* V, 15:593, 1987.
4. Marty R: Experience with a new flexible hysteroscope, *Int J Gynecol Obstet* 27:97, 1988.
5. Marty R: Presentation d'un hysteroscope de la troisième generation: le Fujinon flexible system 2000, *Congres de la Federation des Gynecologues Obstetriciens Francais* 17:54, 1988.
6. Mussuto P: The challenges of flexibility in hysteroscopy: its diagnostic and therapeutic contributions in obstetrics and gynecology, Future prospects, Thesis PA 060032, 1993. Faculté de Médecine Broussais, Hotel-Dieu, France, 1993.
7. Lignary C, Sahel J: *Endoscopie Digestive Pratique.* Pissin, Ed: 1988.

Chapter 5

NURSING IMPLICATIONS FOR HYSTEROSCOPY IN AN OUTPATIENT SETTING

Suzanne O. Tempesta
Maureen P. Spencer

With the introduction of outpatient hysteroscopy, the office nurse faces new challenges within the ambulatory gynecology practice. Office hysteroscopy can be performed using either a flexible or a rigid endoscope, and nursing care remains consistent with either type of instrumentation. Nursing interventions can be assigned to one of three categories: patient care, office preparation/physician assistance, and equipment maintenance. Nurses play a principal role in facilitating this process by helping to provide a well-tolerated, low-risk procedure that will provide vital information concerning a patient's intrauterine condition. This information was previously attainable only in the operating room.

PATIENT EDUCATION

Direct patient care focuses on patient education and observation. The patient will have questions that should be addressed before, during, and after the procedure. Attending to these needs will lessen a patient's anxiety about undergoing hysteroscopy in the office.

Purpose for the procedure

Although the physician will have initially explained the reason for performing an office hysteroscopy, patients may be unclear about these indications when they call to schedule an appointment. The nurse should take the time, before the procedure, to review with each patient exactly why this procedure has been recommended. Depending on history, symptoms, and/or diagnosis, the patient should fully understand what information the doctor expects to obtain from the pro-

cedure. For example, if a woman has experienced recurrent miscarriage, she should understand that the purpose of the office hysteroscopy is to rule out uterine pathology, such as submucous myomata, endometrial polyps, uterine septa, or adhesions, that might contribute to spontaneous abortion. Most often office hysteroscopy will be used as a diagnostic tool. In this case, it should be clear to the patient that no treatment will be performed at the time of the procedure. Alternatively, if the physician plans to offer treatment during office hysteroscopy (i.e., polypectomy), the nurse should make sure the patient is aware of the risks and benefits of such intervention.

Positioning

Once the patient understands why hysteroscopy has been recommended, a brief explanation of what will occur during the procedure is usually helpful. The nurse should emphasize what the patient will experience rather than the activity that will take place around her. She should be informed that she will be asked to undress from the waist down and that she will remain adequately draped throughout the procedure. Let her know that she will be placed on the examination table in the lithotomy position, with which most patients are familiar from previous gynecologic examinations.

Preparation of the cervix

As the procedure begins, the physician will insert a vaginal speculum to visualize the cervix. Once the speculum is in place, the patient will initially feel a cold disinfectant solution being applied to the cervix. Reviewing this step before beginning the procedure gives the nurse an opportunity to check for allergies to topical solutions such as povidone-iodine. On occasion, the physician will need to apply a tenaculum to the cervix to pass the hysteroscope. If this is the case, the patient should be warned to expect a pinching or "bee sting" sensation. If the cervix is unusually stenotic, it may be necessary to use cervical dilators to ensure adequate dilatation. During this portion of the procedure, the patient can expect menstrual-like cramps. Some physicians will opt to administer a paracervical block before inserting the hysteroscope. This block will feel like a pinch followed by a burning sensation that will last for a few seconds. You may find the use of a tenaculum, cervical block, or dilators more common when using the rigid hysteroscope.

Discomfort/premedication

Once the cervix is prepared, the physician will attempt to pass the hysteroscope through the cervix into the uterine cavity. At this point many patients will experience some uterine cramping. While some patients report virtually no discomfort, a small number find it quite painful, and the majority report mild to moderate cramps. Patients may be offered an analgesic such as ibuprofen an hour before the procedure to lessen the discomfort. Assure the patient that if she finds the procedure intolerable, it can be discontinued at any time, with rapid relief of symptoms.

Distention media

Throughout the procedure, the uterus is flushed with a sterile nonviscous solution such as lactated Ringer's or saline. The solution flows directly out through the vagina; thus the patient may feel warm wetness coming from the vagina. She should be advised in advance to expect this sensation so that she does not mistakenly suspect that she is bleeding.

Anatomy

If video equipment is available, some patients will be distracted by, as well as interested in, seeing what the doctor sees. The nurse can help by identifying anatomy during this phase, freeing the physician to concentrate on evaluating the endocervix and uterine cavity.

Post-procedure instructions

After having visualized the entire uterine cavity, the physician will first remove the hysteroscope and then the speculum. The patient should be instructed to remain supine for several minutes before attempting to sit up. Inform her that some individuals experience dizziness, flushing, or nausea but that these symptoms resolve quickly after the procedure is finished. Vital signs should be assessed if the patient appears to be in distress during or after the hysteroscopy. If the patient fully understands what she may experience during the hysteroscopy, she is less likely to be anxious or fearful, thus making the procedure more comfortable for everyone. Final discharge instructions should be given when the pa-

tient is fully recovered. There are no dietary or activity restrictions. Because the cervix is dilated to only 3 to 5 mm, it is not necessary to prohibit the use of tampons or restrict douching or intercourse. She should expect a watery, brown discharge throughout the day as the remainder of the flushing solution and povidone-iodine drains from the cervix. Some light spotting is also not unusual. The patient must be told to notify her physician if she experiences a worsening of symptoms (severe abdominal pain, heavy or bright red bleeding, or a temperature elevation greater than 100° F).

OFFICE PREPARATION AND PHYSICIAN ASSISTANCE

Preparing the examination room for office hysteroscopy can be accomplished quickly and efficiently by setting up three work areas: one for the physician, one for the nurse, and one for the patient. Properly equipping each of these areas will ensure a successful procedure, as well as easier cleanup and room turnover. The box below summarizes the ancillary equipment needed for office hysteroscopy.

Patient area

The patient will be positioned on the examining table. One hospital underpad or "chux" should be placed under the patient's buttocks, one on the end of the table, extending halfway down the front of the table, and one on the step of the table to absorb any extra flow from the saline used for insufflation (Fig. 5-1). If a lengthy procedure is anticipated or

---

Equipment and materials needed to perform office hysteroscopy

Patient area

Hospital underpads
Drape

Physician area

Speculum
8-inch cotton-tipped applicators (3)
Povidone-iodine
Tenaculum
Forceps
Cervical dilators
Sterile gloves
Face shield
Gown

Nurse area

Hysteroscope
500 ml sterile saline
60-ml syringe
15-gauge needle
Sterile specimen cup
IV tubing
Scissors
Alcohol swab

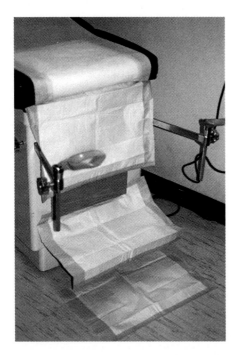

Fig. 5-1. Preparation of examination for hysteroscopy.

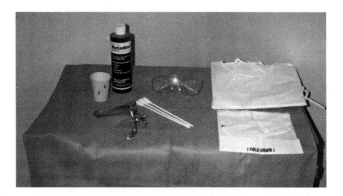

Fig. 5-2. Setup for the physician's work area.

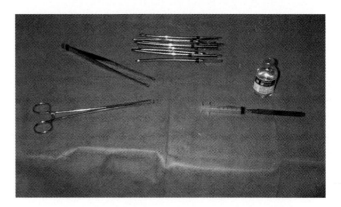

Fig. 5-3. Optional instruments used in hysteroscopy.

if a 5-mm hysteroscope will be used, extra underpads should be placed on the floor in front of the examination table to catch overflow. Each patient is provided a drape.

Physician area

A small table should be placed within easy reach of the physician, who will be seated at the end of the examination table. Place a speculum, three 8-inch cotton-tipped applicators saturated with povidone-iodine, a pair of sterile gloves, a protective gown, and a face shield or goggles on this table (Fig. 5-2). Certain instruments should be available, although they may not be used in each case (Fig. 5-3). A tenaculum may be needed to grasp the cervix and allow for easier passage of the hysteroscope. A postcoital forcep (also known as a Singley tissue forcep) may be used to add rigidity to the flexible end of the hysteroscope as it is passed through the cervix. Cervical dilation may be required, in which case a set of dilators sized in half-millimeter increments from 1 to 8 (1 mm, 1.5 mm, 2 mm, 2.5 mm, etc.) should be adequate. A 6-ml syringe with a 22-gauge, 3½-inch spinal needle filled with 1% lidocaine hydrochloride should be available if requested for cervical anesthesia. Finally, if the physician routinely uses a tenaculum, it is advisable to have instruments such as a large needle driver, chromic suture, and forceps available to repair cervical tears.

Nurse area

The nurse's work area should be large enough to hold the hysteroscope and materials for insufflation, including a 500-ml bottle of sterile saline, a 60-ml syringe with a Luer-Lok tip, a 15-gauge needle, a sterile specimen cup, basic IV solution tubing (or extension tubing), a pair of scissors, a

package of sterile gauze, and an alcohol swab (Fig. 5-4). The uterine cavity is flushed continuously during the procedure to clear the visual field and distend the cavity slightly. The 60-ml syringe, filled with saline and attached to the hysteroscope with IV tubing, is one method used to manually insufflate the cavity. The IV tubing should have a port at least 12 inches away from the point at which it attaches to the hysteroscope so that the nurse has some space in which to maneuver and so that the physician looking through the eyepiece is not crowded by the insufflation setup. A needle smaller than 15 gauge may provide too much resistance to the individual who is manually flushing the cavity and therefore may not allow for adequate distention.

As you become familiar with preparing the examination room for hysteroscopy, you will likely establish a routine that is thorough and efficient. One step-by-step method is offered below:

Place one underpad at the end of the examination table and under the patient.

Place one underpad on the step and floor if necessary.

Leave a patient drape on the table.

Saturate three 8-inch cotton-tipped applicators with povidone-iodine and set aside on the physician's work table.

Open one package of sterile gloves and one speculum and place on work table.

Place a protective gown and face shield on this table.

Have a tenaculum, forceps, and dilators available.

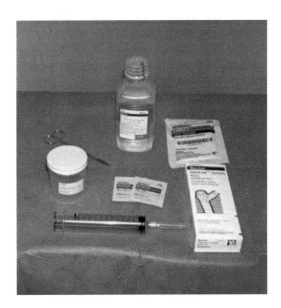

Fig. 5-4. Setup for nurse's work area.

At the nurse's work area:

Open a 500-ml bottle of sterile saline.

Fill a sterile specimen cup with saline.

Fill the 60-ml syringe from this cup.

Refill the specimen cup and set aside.

Attach the 15-gauge needle to the syringe.

Open the IV tubing set and clamp it closed (tubing that extends beyond the clamp can be cut off for easier handling).

Swab the distal port of the IV tubing with alcohol.

Insert the needle and syringe into the IV tubing at the distal port.*

Attach the IV tubing to the hysteroscope at the channel post.

While the hysteroscopy is under way, the nurse is often responsible for providing uterine distention while also observing the patient's tolerance of the procedure. With the 60-ml syringe and IV tubing, distention begins when the hysteroscope reaches the internal os and is adequately maintained using manual pressure without too much or too little resistance. A thorough evaluation can be completed, often using less than one full 60-ml syringe. If more distention medium is needed, the syringe can be refilled during the examination or more than one syringe can be prepared in advance.

After the examination, the nurse should ensure that the patient is stable before reprocessing the hysteroscope.

EQUIPMENT PROCESSING AND MAINTENANCE

The two principal reasons for proper equipment maintenance are to maximize the useful life of the endoscope and minimize the chance of infection.

*If video equipment is being used, the color on the camera must be readjusted by "white balancing." Before attaching the IV tubing, place the camera on the eyepiece. Place the tip of the endoscope 1 to 2 cm from a sterile gauze, focus, and press the white balance button until the flashing light becomes steady. The scope and camera are now ready to use.

Infection related to endoscopic procedures is caused by both endogenous and exogenous microorganisms. Colonizing microorganisms of the vaginal tract can enter the uterus or bloodstream as a consequence of hysteroscopy. Exogenous microorganisms may be associated with contaminated endoscopic equipment, or contamination from the environment or health care workers involved in the procedure. Cleaning and high-level disinfection or sterilization of the hysteroscope is essential to prevent intrauterine or bloodstream infections.

HYSTEROSCOPE REPROCESSING PROCEDURES

Endoscopic instruments must be meticulously cleaned before disinfection or sterilization. The methods employed to achieve these conditions should be detailed in policies and procedures, preferably developed in collaboration with the facility's infection control committee.

Disinfection of the hysteroscope

When developing and choosing a disinfection procedure, it is important to consider the desired level of germicidal action. A hysteroscope is classified as a "semicritical" medical device because it comes into contact with mucous membranes.[1] High-level disinfection is recommended for semicritical items because it inactivates all vegetative bacteria, mycobacteria, fungi, and viruses. However, it does not necessarily inactivate all bacterial endospores.

The disinfectant of choice is one that will neither be toxic to personnel nor cause damage to the scope, and its action will not be significantly decreased by the presence of organic matter. Unfortunately, many high-level disinfectants do not meet all of these criteria and are not recommended for use on endoscopes. Iodophors, hypochlorite, quarternary ammonium compounds, and phenolics are not recommended disinfectants, either because of their corrosiveness or their inadequate disinfection properties.

Other factors that affect the efficacy of germicides include the type and number of microorganisms, the concentration and exposure time of the disinfectant, the temperature, and the pH of the disinfection process.

Chemical germicides

Chemical germicides (high-level disinfectants/cold sterilants) intended for use on critical and semicritical devices are subject to a premarket review of safety and efficacy by the Food and Drug Administration (FDA). Manufacturer's recommendations for dilution and immersion times are included on product labels. To achieve high-level disinfection, most disinfectants require an immersion time of less than 1 hour, while cold sterilization requires a more extended immersion period, usually 6 to 8 hours.

Glutaraldehyde 2%* is a chemical germicide indicated for high-level disinfection and cold sterilization and in the

*Cidex, Johnson & Johnson Medical, Inc; Metricide, Metrex Research Corp.

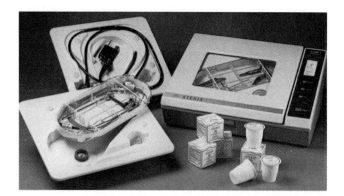

Fig. 5-5. Steris automated endoscopic reprocessing.

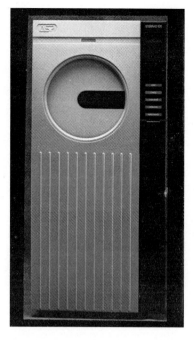

Fig. 5-6. Sterrad vapor-phase hydrogen peroxide chamber.

past has been the most frequently used chemical for this purpose. The Occupational Safety and Health Administration (OSHA) has issued ceiling limits on the permissible level of glutaraldehyde in the air at 0.2 ppm because it may cause irritation of the respiratory tracts of staff members when concentrations are above this limit.[2] Therefore, it must be used in properly ventilated areas, and care should be taken to limit manipulation of the liquid by personnel during use. Many clinics and offices do not have adequate ventilation to remove toxic fumes from the air. Consequently, staff members may experience skin and nasal mucosa irritation, which can ultimately result in respiratory ailments, headache, rashes, and contact irritation.[3] In addition, endoscopes that have been disinfected in glutaraldehyde have the potential to cause adverse outcomes in patients, such as chemical colitis from absorption of glutaraldehyde when the endoscopes are not adequately rinsed.[4]

Additional practices that are advised when using glutaraldehyde include pH monitoring, especially when highly acidic detergents are used in precleaning and may not have been thoroughly rinsed off, and neutralizing the glutaraldehyde before disposal to minimize staff exposure. Unless restricted by state and/or local sewer authorities, glutaraldehyde can be discarded, without first neutralizing it, by flushing it down the drain with water.

Staff members need to take additional safety precautions when working with glutaraldehyde. These precautions include the use of nitrile rubber, butyl rubber, or polyethylene gloves. Latex, neoprene, and polyvinyl chloride gloves are not recommended. Additionally, eye protection and gowns suitable for protection against splashing chemicals should be worn.

Six percent hydrogen peroxide/85% phosphoric acid* solution was previously approved as a high-level disinfectant/cold sterilant, but has been removed from the market and is undergoing a change in formulation. Although it is a potent antimicrobial agent, it can damage rubbers and plastics and may corrode copper, zinc, and brass.[5]

Ethylene oxide gas sterilization (ETO-CFC)

Fiberscopes can withstand ethylene oxide gas (ETO) sterilization provided the scope is physically clean and thoroughly dried before the cycle. Restricted regulations related to the use of chlorofluorocarbons (CFCs), increased emissions-level controls in various states, and regulation as an occupational hazard have prompted hospitals to examine their use of ETO-CFC sterilization. Alternatives include combinations of ETO with CO_2, hydrochlorofluorocarbons (HCFCs), and the use of 100% ETO.

Low-temperature sterilization technologies

There has been an increase in low-temperature sterilization technology. All techniques have advantages and disadvantages, but these processes are emerging as safer alternatives to chemical germicides.

Peracetic acid† (Fig. 5-5) is a mixture of acetic acid, hydrogen peroxide, and water. An automated endoscopic reprocessing system is available that dilutes 35% peracetic acid to a final concentration of 0.2% and adds a buffer and an anticorrosive agent. It is approved for use with hysterofiberscopes by the scope manufacturer. The precleaning process is still required, but the high agitation action of the disinfection cycle removes residue and debris within the channels. The length of the sterilization cycle with the automated machine is 30 minutes.

Hydrogen peroxide gas–plasma‡ (Fig. 5-6) is a new low-temperature sterilization technique. Items are placed into a sterilization chamber, a vacuum is created, and the solution (58% hydrogen peroxide) is injected automatically to sur-

*Endospore, Glove Medical.

†Steris System 1, Steris Corp.

‡Sterrad, Advanced Sterilization Products, Division of Johnson & Johnson Medical, Inc.

round the items to be sterilized. At the end of the sterilization cycle, the active components recombine to form oxygen and vaporized water. There are no toxic residues so aeration is not required. The complete sterilization cycle takes an hour. Items cannot be wrapped in cellulose (paper) or linen, and liquids cannot be processed. The system is indicated for metal and nonmetal instruments, and for many heat- and moisture-sensitive instruments. Rigid endoscopes with channels or lumens no longer than 31 cm (12 inches) or narrower than 6 mm (one quarter inch) can be subjected to this process but, at present, hysterofiberscopes cannot. An accessory to facilitate sterilization of devices with long narrow lumens, such as flexible endoscopes, is available in countries worldwide but is awaiting approval by the FDA for use in the United States.

This low-temperature sterilization process requires precleaning of medical devices. Laboratory tests confirm broad-spectrum activity against vegetative bacteria, bacterial spores, fungi, and viruses.

Plasma sterilization,* which uses a system that combines peracetic acid with hydrogen and oxygen and exposes the solution to an electromagnetic field, is another new low-temperature sterilization technique. This plasma system penetrates packaging material (Tyvek/Mylar, woven wraps, Paper/Mylar), has no corrosive effects, and is safe for the environment and personnel. Cycle time depends on load (up to 6 hours) and no aeration is necessary. This process is ideal for heat-sensitive items, but because it is so new, its effectiveness has not been verified in peer-review studies.

Other techniques for low-temperature sterilization are vaporized hydrogen peroxide and ozone. These are the newest emerging technologies and currently have not been approved for use on medical devices in the United States.

Steam sterilization

Because of their heat stability, many rigid hysteroscopes can be reprocessed using an autoclave. Manufacturers should recommend whether this option is appropriate for their product. Currently, no flexible hysteroscope is compatible with this method of sterilization.

REPROCESSING PROCEDURES

Precleaning procedure

The precleaning procedure should include the following steps:

1. Immediately after the procedure, wipe the insertion tube with a gauze.
2. When using syringes, alternate irrigating the channel with clean water and a cleaning solution. The cleaning solution should be a detergent that contains enzymes that digest organic material and protein on contact within a 3- to 5-minute period.

3. Perform the leak test procedure detailed by the manufacturer of the hysterofiberscope.

Cleaning procedure

To clean the instrument, perform the following steps:

1. Immerse the entire instrument in the enzymatic solution and scrub the external surfaces.
2. Remove the scope and place it in an immersible bin of clean water; rinse thoroughly.
3. Insert the channel cleaning brush through the channel post and brush the entire instrument channel.
4. Alternate irrigating the channel with clean water and cleaning solution to remove debris loosened during the brushing procedure.
5. Finish with a thorough rinse of clean water.
6. Blow plenty of air into the channel to remove water. Dry all external surfaces of the instrument to prevent water from diluting the disinfectant solution.

Liquid high-level disinfection procedure for flexible and rigid hysteroscopes

The procedure for using liquid disinfectants with flexible and rigid hysteroscopes is as follows:

1. Immerse the hysteroscope in the disinfectant immersion bin and pump disinfectant through the channel with a syringe.
2. Allow the scope to remain in the solution for the recommended immersion time.
3. Following disinfection, remove the scope and irrigate the channel with water until thoroughly rinsed.
4. Rinse the outside of the scope and place it in an immersion bin filled with water. Allow it to soak to remove all disinfectant.
5. If clean (tap) water is used, the rinse must be followed with 70% alcohol rinse because tap water may inoculate the inside lumen of the channel with waterborne microorganisms that could incubate.
6. Remove the scope and place it on a clean, dry surface.
7. Run air through the channel until all moisture has been expelled and the channel is dry.
8. Wipe the outside surface of the scope until dry.
9. Store in a manner to prevent recontamination or damage. Never store in the case in foam material because fungus is known to grow in these areas.

Sterilization of flexible and rigid hysteroscopes

Cold sterilization. Cold sterilization of flexible and rigid hysteroscopes should proceed as follows:

1. Perform the cleaning procedure as outlined above.
2. Perform the disinfection procedure steps as outlined above.
3. The scope must be immersed in the sterilant solution according to the manufacturer's recommendations but must *not exceed* 10 hours.

*Plazlyte.

4. After four extended immersion periods, the scope must be aerated to reduce the level of internal humidity. Leave the ethylene oxide (ETO) cap attached during aeration for 15 hours.

ETO sterilization. ETO sterilization of hysteroscopes should be completed as follows:

1. Perform the precleaning procedure as outlined above.
2. Be sure the scope is thoroughly dried before the cycle.
3. The ETO cap must be securely on the light guide connector and must remain in place throughout sterilization and aeration.

Autoclaving rigid hysteroscopes

If the endoscope manufacturer recommends steam sterilization for the product, the following parameters can be used for temperature and exposure time once the instrument has been thoroughly cleaned:

Gravity-displacement steam sterilization
Wrapped   270 to 275° F for 10 to 15 minutes
             250 to 254° F for 15 to 30 minutes
Unwrapped   270° F for 3 minutes
Prevacuum steam sterilization
Wrapped   270 to 275° F for 3 to 4 minutes
Unwrapped   270° F for 3 to 4 minutes
Steam-flush pressure pulse steam sterilization
Wrapped   250 to 254° F for 20 minutes
Unwrapped   270 to 275° F for 3 to 4 minutes

Processing endoscopic accessory equipment

Instruments, such as biopsy forceps, that penetrate mucous barriers are considered "critical" items and therefore must be sterilized before use. Biopsy forceps may be steam sterilized or purchased as disposable items.

Adverse occurrences

Hospitals, offices, and clinics in which endoscopic procedures are performed should have in place policies and procedures that specify the monitoring and reporting of adverse occurrences resulting from the procedure. Safety, infection control, and risk management programs are usually available to assist whenever epidemiologic evidence suggests infection transmission by endoscopes, adverse toxic effects from disinfectants, sterilization failure, or sterilizer malfunction. Numerous infectious outbreaks have been reported because of endoscopic procedures. The FDA[7] has issued a final rule requiring "device user facilities" to report adverse events such as deaths, serious illnesses, and injuries related to medical devices. Any person who processes a device by chemical, physical, or biologic means is considered a device manufacturer and must comply with manufacturing standards. In addition, the Joint Commission on Accreditation of Healthcare Organizations (JCAHO) requires written policies on the reprocessing of items including precleaning, wrapping, and sterilization procedures and quality assurance monitoring.

Establishing policies and procedures for reprocessing

Institutional resources
Environmental barriers
Space
Instrument compatability
Time
Staff
Number of handlers
Quality assurance documentation
Cost

The box outlines issues to be considered when establishing policies and procedures for reprocessing hysteroscopes.

Reprocessing facilities and space

A designated area should be assigned for the reprocessing procedures that is separate from direct care areas. There should be a large sink to clean the scope, sufficient counter space for the immersion bins, and an area to dry the scope, irrigate it with alcohol, and blow air into its channels. If glutaraldehyde is going to be used, discuss ventilation requirements with safety consultants.

CONCLUSION

Proper care and maintenance of the hysteroscope will extend its life and ensure safety and performance. It is important that those people who will handle the equipment, thoroughly understand the manufacturer's recommendations before use. Adequately designed work areas to reprocess endoscopic equipment and well-trained staff members are essential to provide safe endoscopic procedures to patients.

REFERENCES

1. Spaulding EH: Chemical disinfection of medical and surgical materials. In Lawrence CA, Block SS, Eds: *Disinfection, sterilization, and preservation,* ed 3, Philadelphia, 1968, Lea & Febiger.
2. Occupational Safety and Health Administration: Air contaminants, *Federal Register* 54:2332-464, 1989.
3. Center for Disease Control: Symptoms of irritation associated with exposure to glutaraldehyde—Colorado, *MMWR* 36:190-1, 1987.
4. Jonas G, Mahoney A, Murray J, Gerther S: Chemical colitis due to endoscope cleaning solutions: a mimic of pseudomembranous colitis, *Gastroenterology* 95:1403-8, 1988.
5. Block SS: Peroxygen compounds. In Block SS, Ed: *Disinfection, sterilization, and preservation,* ed 4, Philadelphia, 1991, Lea & Febiger.
6. Association for the Advancement of Medical Instrumentation: Designing, testing, and labeling reusable medical devices for reprocessing in healthcare facilities: a guide for device manufacturers, *TIR No 12,* 1994, The Association.
7. Department of Health and Human Services, Food and Drug Administration: Medical devices: medical device, user facility, distributor, and manufacturer reporting, certification, and registration, proposed rule 21, CFR parts 803 and 807, *Federal Register* 56:60024-30, 1991.

Chapter 6

UTERINE DISTENTION

Misty Blanchette Porter
John R. Brumsted

Establishing a panoramic view within the uterine cavity is of utmost importance for both diagnostic and operative hysteroscopy. Appropriate identification of both normal structures and pathologic conditions within the potential space of the uterine cavity depends largely on the ability to obtain a clear operative view. The type of distention medium chosen rests primarily on the goal of the surgery, be it diagnostic or therapeutic, the instrumentation chosen, and physician preference. Certain procedures and instrumentation present natural choices for one medium over another. Although Dr. Gimpleson in Chapter 10 has described several therapeutic procedures that can be done using office hysteroscopy, it generally is a diagnostic procedure. Because no electricity is being used in diagnostic hysteroscopy, there is no need for hypotonic solutions. As well, most diagnostic hysteroscopy will not be performed while the patient has moderate to heavy vaginal bleeding; otherwise, either continuous-flow hysteroscopy or viscous solutions, such as dextran 70, would be required. More than 95% of office hysteroscopies are performed with either CO_2 or isotonic nonviscous solutions such as normal saline or lactated Ringer's solution. This chapter will present a discussion of the indications, method of use, limitations, and potential complications of each distending medium used for either diagnostic or therapeutic hysteroscopy.

DISTENTION MEDIA FOR DIAGNOSTIC HYSTEROSCOPY

Carbon dioxide

Carbon dioxide is a colorless gas that is useful for diagnostic hysteroscopy. Its relative ease of use makes it ideal for office hysteroscopy, and it is safe when used with the proper insufflation apparatus. Lindeman and Mohr,[1] reporting on a collected series of more than 1200 hysteroscopic procedures using CO_2, encountered no serious complications from the gas. Hysteroscopic insufflators are specially designed for and have been widely employed to deliver this medium. These insufflators provide a continuous flow of gas measured in cc/minute, and can adjust the flow rate for a pre-set intrauterine pressure. If the pressure increases, the flow rate drops, minimizing the risk of complications arising from too much insufflated gas or excessively high intrauterine pressure. The recommended maximum flow rate of CO_2 is 100 cc/minute, and the maximum intrauterine pressure is 200 mm Hg.[2] Adequate visualization is usually obtained with a flow rate of 40 to 60 cc/minute and a pressure of 40 to 80 mm Hg.[1]

Laparoscopic insufflators are unsuitable for use with hysteroscopy. They provide CO_2 in liters/minute and at much greater pressures. The complications observed with CO_2 have been largely attributable to the improper selection of insufflation apparatus. Rupture of normal oviducts, hydrosalpinx, and the diaphragm have been reported (9/38). Cardiac arrhythmia and cardiac arrest have also been reported and are presumed to have also resulted from the intravasation of large quantities of CO_2.[1] However, a large margin of safety may exist, as suggested from animal models,[1,3] in which a large quantity of gas directly insufflated into the femoral vein produced few cardiovascular complications. Nevertheless, physicians should adhere to the recommended rates of delivery of the gas, and should use the minimal amount of gas necessary to maintain uterine distention. Patients known to have an atrial septal defect and/or pulmonary hypertension may be at increased risk for CO_2 embolism, and an alternative medium should be considered. In these patients, CO_2 can be shunted from the left atrium to the right atrium.

In a 1991 membership survey, the American Association of Gynecologic Laparoscopists reported the incidence of CO_2 embolism as 0.1/1000 cases of operative hysteroscopy.[4] Although details have not been reported, CO_2 embolism and death have also occurred with the use of CO_2-cooled Nd:YAG laser fibers and artificial sapphire tips.[5-7] Flow rates of CO_2 used to cool the laser fibers and the tips are similar to those delivered via laparoscopic insufflators: 500 to 1000 cc/minute. Several reports of cardiovascular collapse and death as a result of massive CO_2 embolization have prompted the FDA to issue a warning against the use of gas-cooled fibers and tips for intrauterine surgery.[8]

CO_2, however, is an ideal medium for outpatient diagnostic hysteroscopy. It does not clog surgical instruments, it is readily available, and it is well tolerated by the patient under local anesthesia.[1] This finding was corroborated by De Jong et al,[9] who reported on 152 outpatient diagnostic hysteroscopies with CO_2 distention that were successfully completed using a 1% lidocaine paracervical block. Although patients who exhibited "extreme" anxiety were excluded, their population included nulliparous women and patients who had previously undergone cone biopsy. Most of these women described the pain associated with the procedure as acceptable, and 90% found the discomfort no greater than that of menstruation.[9]

Visualization of the uterine cavity with CO_2 has been reported as adequate in a large series.[1] The diagnostic hysteroscope is introduced directly into the endocervical canal without dilation of the cervix, and a continuous flow of CO_2 is provided through tubing by the insufflation device connected to the inflow port on the hysteroscope. The hysteroscope is then advanced under direct visualization as the gas distends the endocervical canal and uterine cavity. The gas seal may be further improved by applying an appropriately sized cervical suction cup or a four-pronged tenaculum.[10,11]

Examining the patient in the follicular phase and gentle manipulation of the instruments may both improve the quality of the view and minimize bleeding and the amount of mucus obscuring the field. Because of its lower index of refraction, CO_2 offers a wider field of view and a reduction in the magnification needed compared with liquid media. However, CO_2 bubbles can mix with blood and form a foam that obscures the operative field. It also tends to flatten the endometrium, concealing pathology. Reflux of the gas may limit visualization in multiparous patients and those who have had a cone biopsy. These characteristics make it a poor choice for operative procedures.

Normal saline or lactated Ringer's solution

An alternative to CO_2 for uterine distention during office hysteroscopy is the use of an isotonic nonviscous solution such as normal saline or lactated Ringer's. The diagnostic

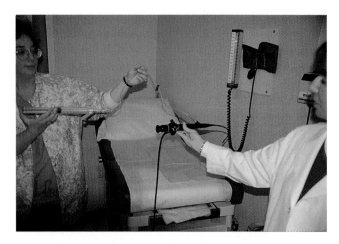

Fig. 6-1. Nonviscous fluid for uterine distention during office hysteroscopy. A 60-ml syringe is filled with normal saline and connected to the working channel of the 3.6-mm flexible hysteroscope via IV tubing. Adequate intrauterine pressure for distention is provided by the assistant. An average of 35 ml is necessary to perform a complete diagnostic hysteroscopy.

hysteroscopic procedure routinely lasts only 2 to 3 minutes, and very little solution is necessary to completely visualize the cervical canal and uterine cavity. Saline or lactated Ringer's is drawn up into a 60-ml syringe and connected to the operative port of the hysteroscope via standard IV tubing (Fig. 6-1). The nursing assistant will slowly push the syringe once the hysteroscope is placed within the cervical canal, thereby dilating the canal. As described with CO_2 insufflation, the hysteroscope is advanced through the cervical canal into the uterine cavity under direct visualization. If an assistant is not available, a 250-cc bag can be hung within an insufflated blood pressure cuff to provide distention. If a rigid hysteroscope is used, it is a good idea to place a paracervical block and use a tenaculum on the anterior lip of the cervix. If a 3.6-mm flexible hysteroscope is used with nonviscous fluid distention, more than 90% of procedures can be performed with no anesthesia or tenaculum.

Most diagnostic hysteroscopies can be performed with less than 60 ml of fluid. Rarely will more than 120 to 180 ml be used. This volume is well within the safe limits, even if all of the fluid is absorbed by the patient. Likewise, the limited amount of fluid used does not create a mess in the examination room. When up to 200 ml of fluid is used, the excess fluid exiting the cervix is easily absorbed by placing a pad beneath the patient and another on the floor beneath the hysteroscope (Fig. 6-2).

Unlike CO_2, nonviscous distention solutions neither flatten endometrial tissue nor create mucous bubbles and foaming. On the contrary, normal saline and lactated Ringer's accentuate uterine pathology if the procedure is performed in the early proliferative phase. If performed in the late proliferative or secretory phase, the endometrial lining will absorb

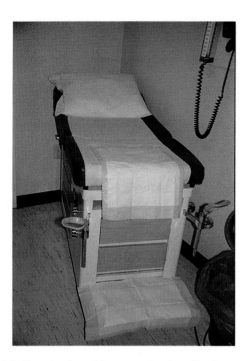

Fig. 6-2. Examination table preparation for office hysteroscopy. A total of three chux are used to collect the fluid used during office hysteroscopy—one under the patient's buttocks and lower back, one under the patient's buttocks and extending down the examination table, and one at the foot of the table.

the solution, making it difficult to identify small lesions such as endometrial polyps.

Dextran 70

Dextran 70, or Hyskon,* is a colorless, viscous, polysaccharide liquid that is optically clear. It comprises a solution of 32% dextran 70 in 10% dextrose in water. Dextran 70 is a mixture of *d*-glucose polymers whose average molecular weight is 70,000 Da and is a product of bacterial polymerization of glucose on the surface of the cell. Hyskon is electrolyte-free, nonconductive, and biodegradable, and is immiscible with blood. These properties make it a valuable tool when the procedure is to be performed during a bleeding episode, and it is a reasonable alternative for both diagnostic and operative procedures with rigid hysteroscopes. It is too viscous to be used with flexible hysteroscopy.

Hyskon is provided in 100-ml bottles. To avoid the formation of bubbles, it should be poured slowly down the side of a sterile container and then aspirated carefully into a 60-ml syringe. It is then flushed through IV extension tubing that has been connected to the inflow port of the hysteroscope. The preflushed instrument is then carefully inserted into the already dilated endocervical canal, and the solution is slowly injected by hand. Again, the best seal is obtained if the endocervical canal is dilated just barely enough to admit the hys-

teroscope. Approximately 5 to 10 ml of Hyskon is required to initially distend the cavity. Once the view is clear, a steady pressure is maintained on the filled syringe. When a pump is used, the maximum pressure should be no greater than 150 mm Hg.

The major disadvantage of Hyskon is that it is sticky and, when dry, tends to harden and crystallize onto the equipment. Immediately after the procedure, the instruments must be soaked in hot water to avoid clogging and the solidification of the dextran within the instrument's operative channels. Stopcock valves on the operative sheaths may jam and require resoaking before use. Additionally, because of its viscous nature, Hyskon cannot be used with instrumentation designed for a continuous flow or with flexible hysteroscopes. Although some authors have described its use with the resectoscope,[12] Hyskon tends to caramelize when exposed to the heat generated by electrosurgical energy, making it a poor choice in this setting.

Usually less than 100 ml of Hyskon is necessary for each procedure. The maximum volume recommended from the manufacturer is 500 ml per case. To limit the potential for complication from intravasation of Hyskon, an alternative strategy is to limit the amount of absorbed dextran to 300 ml. This takes into account a small amount that may be retrieved from the peritoneal cavity by simultaneous suctioning of the cul-de-sac via laparoscopy if this procedure is to be completed for other indications.

Noncardiogenic pulmonary edema has been reported as a complication with the use of much larger volumes of Hyskon (600 to 1200 ml).[13-18] Dextrans are potent plasma expanders, and the pulmonary edema is presumed to be secondary to a marked expansion of the plasma volume. Large–molecular-weight dextran molecules are limited to the intravascular space and markedly increase plasma oncotic pressure.[19] Each gram of dextran 70 will attract approximately 27 ml of water.[20] Therefore, for each 100 ml of Hyskon intravasated, the plasma volume is expanded by 860 ml.[20] Fluid and electrolytes are drawn intravascularly from the interstitial and third-space compartments. Thus the intravasation of 300 ml of Hyskon could result in an increase in the plasma volume by almost 3000 ml, causing an intravascular volume overload. Furthermore, this effect is long lasting because the plasma half-life of large–molecular-weight dextrans is several days.[21]

Another less uniformly accepted theory on the cause of pulmonary edema is a direct toxic effect of the dextran molecules on pulmonary capillaries.[15,16,18] The mechanism of insult to the capillaries is presumed to be similar to the drug-induced noncardiogenic pulmonary edema reported with methadone, heroin, ritodrine, and salicylates, and has been reported with the use other dextrans (i.e., dextran 40).[15,22] This effect is thought to increase capillary leakage, thereby contributing further to, and accelerating the development of, pulmonary edema. However, this direct toxic effect has not been demonstrated in animal models.[23]

*Pharmacia, Hyskon Division, Piscataway, NJ.

Intravascular coagulopathy,[13,17,18,24] renal insufficiency or failure,[25] and rhabdomyolysis[13] have been reported in association with noncardiogenic pulmonary edema as a complication of dextran intravasation. Frequently, presenting symptoms in these patients included frothy fluid from the endotracheal tube, respiratory distress and hemoptysis in the recovery room, bleeding from IV sites and the vagina, and bilateral patchy infiltrates on chest radiograph. Almost uniformly, arterial blood gases in these patients revealed mild to moderate hypoxemia, a marked decrease in hemoglobin, platelets and fibrinogen, and an elevation in the prothrombin and partial thromboplastin times.

Dextrans were previously used as an alternative agent to heparin as a thromboprophylactic agent. Dextrans coat both endothelial cells and platelets and decrease platelet adhesiveness to endothelial cells. They also may alter fibrin clot formation and make it more susceptible to lysis. Additionally, by markedly increasing plasma volume, they dilute and reduce the concentration of fibrinogen, factors V, VIII, and IX, and the factor VIII–von Willebrand complex.[25]

In laboratory animals, dextrans can induce oliguric renal failure.[19] Because of their large molecular weight, they are poorly cleared from the blood. Although smaller polymers can be excreted renally, dextrans greater than 50,000 Da are cleared largely by the reticuloendothelial system. Moreover, dextran 40 infusion has been associated with acute renal failure when administered to patients postoperatively.[25,26] A prerequisite for the development of renal failure in association with the use of dextrans appears to be severe constriction of the renal artery.[19] This condition lowers glomerular perfusion pressure and, combined with an elevated plasma oncotic pressure, may induce renal insufficiency. Thus patients with obstructive vascular disease may be at increased risk for the development of renal failure in association with the intravasation of dextrans. Furthermore, dextrans can be precipitated within the renal tubules, forming casts that can lead to mechanical obstruction.[19]

Brandt et al[13] reported on one case of rhabdomyolysis associated with pulmonary disease and coagulopathy after a hysteroscopic treatment of Asherman's syndrome. Approximately 550 ml of Hyskon was intravasated under manual pressure during the course of the 30-minute procedure. In addition to the development of respiratory distress and a coagulopathy, the patient was noted to have a 12-fold increase in her serum creatine kinase level during a 24-hour period. The hyperoncotic state associated with the intravasation of dextrans has been associated with rhabdomyolysis in an experimental model as well, and was said to be largely responsible for the elevation of serum creatine kinase in this patient.

Dextrans have been associated with factitious laboratory findings.[25] They can falsely elevate blood glucose levels and make it more difficult to measure total serum protein and bilirubin concentrations. Additionally, they may cause errors in blood cross-matching if completed by enzyme methods. This situation increases the likelihood for mismatched blood transfusions if the type and screen are acquired after the intravasation of large quantities of dextrans.

Treatment for the complications associated with the absorption of large quantities of Hyskon involves diuresis and respiratory support; patients sometimes also require ventilatory support. Diuresis may be initiated with furosemide, but in cases with intractable pulmonary edema and renal failure, plasmapheresis should be considered.[19] Dialysis is insufficient for therapy. Although the coagulopathy associated with dextran use may be largely corrected with diuresis, the patient may require transfusion, especially where there is overt bleeding.

Hyskon use has been associated with an idiosyncratic anaphylactoid reaction. Large–molecular–weight dextrans are known to be immunogenic. Even with no prior exposure to Hyskon, the patient may respond with anaphylactic shock. The reported incidence of anaphylaxis in response to dextrans is approximately 1/10,000.[27] Ahmed et al[27] reported on three cases of severe anaphylactic reactions in response to Hyskon. In all their patients, the reaction was delayed approximately 10 minutes following exposure, and all patients received less than 100 ml of Hyskon. This reaction is thought to be linked to histamine release and may be attributable to sensitization resulting from exposure to naturally occurring antigens such as commercial sugar, which is frequently contaminated with dextrans, and oral bacteria, which metabolize beet sugar to dextrans. Another source of antigen exposure is through cross reaction with polysaccharides of bacteria: streptococci, pneumococci, and *Salmonella typhosa*.[28] Skin tests are of little value in diagnosing and preventing severe reactions because dextran sensitivity is not mediated by immunoglobulin E.[29] Atopic patients do not appear to be at increased risk.[27] The Hyskon infusion should be immediately discontinued once anaphylaxis is suspected. Treatment involves resuscitation with intravenous or intratracheal epinephrine, 0.5 mg given every 5 to 10 minutes as needed. Hydrocortisone should be administered for serious or prolonged reactions, with its major role being primarily to prevent the redevelopment of symptoms of anaphylaxis.

Nonviscous solutions

Hypotonic. Nonviscous, hypotonic solutions, such as glycine, and sorbitol/mannitol solutions are readily available, inexpensive, and nonconducive. These properties make them ideal for operative hysteroscopic procedures. The complications that arise are due largely to the absorption and intravasation of large volumes of these hypotonic fluids, leading to water intoxication, hypervolemia, and hyponatremia.

Glycine. Glycine is a simple amino acid that is supplied in 3-liter bags as a 1.5% solution with water. It is hypoosmolar (with an osmolality of 200 mOsm/L), nonhemolytic, nonimmunogenic, and electrolyte-free. Experience with the endoscopic use of glycine solutions stems largely from the urologic literature; it has been used as an irrigant for transurethral prostatic resection (TURP) procedures since the 1940s. Water intoxication or pulmonary edema has been reported at a rate of 1.4/1000 hysteroscopic procedures,[4] which is comparable to the rate of 2% described for TURP procedures.[21] It is imperative to keep precise track of the amount of distention fluid used and reclaimed. A closed collection system consisting of a drape placed under the buttocks with an attached pocket should be used. Suction tubing is then applied to the port on the pocket and connected to canister suction. Using this method, fluid balance should then be assessed every 10 to 15 minutes.

The glycine distention medium is delivered to a continuous-flow resectoscope or a multichanneled operative hysteroscope through cystoscopy tubing. The hysteroscope and tubing are first flushed free of air and then, under direct visualization, the hysteroscope is introduced into the pre-dilated cervix and advanced slowly into the uterine cavity. A clear view is then obtained by opening the outflow port of the hysteroscope and allowing blood and debris to be flushed out of the cavity. This process may be hastened, and air bubbles and small pieces of debris may be cleared, by applying manual suction to a ureteral catheter (6F) placed through the operative channel of the hysteroscope.

Traditionally, adequate uterine distention was obtained by elevating the bags of glycine from 60 to 150 cm above the level of the patient's heart. This direct gravity flow system allowed for sufficient visualization but did not provide any method for accurately assessing the achieved intrauterine pressure. Vulgaropulos et al[30] determined that intrauterine pressures of 230 mm Hg could be created with both a tight cervical seal and a closed outflow valve of the hysteroscope with 8 feet of pump pressure. These pressure levels far exceed the maximum pressure of 75 to 100 mm Hg[30,31] needed to complete most operative cases, and markedly increase the chance for excessive intravasation of fluid. In fact, they reported on one case in which 900 ml of fluid was absorbed when the outflow valve was inadvertently left closed for approximately 10 minutes. For this reason, pump infusion systems have come into favor. The absorption of excessive fluid can be minimized if the pressure within the uterine cavity is precisely maintained at the mean blood pressure level. At pressures lower than this, bleeding will occur into the cavity during the operative procedure, obscuring visualization. At pressures higher than mean blood pressure, there will be retrograde flow into the systemic circulation. With the pump system, as the preset level is reached, the delivery of fluid is progressively slowed.[32]

Liquid distention medium is intravasated from the uterine cavity into the uterine vasculature through transected vascular channels. Although a transtubal and peritoneal absorption mechanism has also been proposed, it likely contributes little to the total absorbed fluid volume in cases that do not involve uterine perforation. In fact, Seigler and Kemmann[2] and Siegler and Valle[33] reported that in patients who went directly to laparotomy following hysteroscopy, only 50 to 200 ml of solution was found in the cul-de-sac.[2,34] However, in cases where uterine perforation is suspected and there is a sizable fluid deficit, the patient may benefit from diagnostic laparoscopy and the suctioning of intraperitoneal fluid. Perforation in itself can be associated with the intravasation of large fluid volumes.[30]

In September 1993, Arieff and Ayus[35] reported on several cases of hyponatremic encephalopathy as a complication of endometrial ablation, including one fatality. This is a previously well-described phenomenon, and is known as "post-TURP syndrome" in urologic literature. It is a constellation of symptoms associated with the absorption of large volumes of hypo-osmotic distention medium. Patients present with bradycardia, and frequently hypertension, followed by hypotension, nausea, vomiting, headache, visual disturbances, agitation, confusion, and lethargy. These symptoms are the result of hypervolemia, dilutional hyponatremia, and decreased plasma osmolarity.[36,37] If left untreated, the syndrome may progress to seizures, coma, cardiovascular collapse, and death.[21,26]

Ghanem and Ward[36] showed that the mean drop in serum osmolality was significant in patients who were symptomatic. Under normal circumstances, sodium and its associated ions account for the majority of plasma osmolarity. Therefore a drop in serum sodium concentration is reflected by a drop in serum osmolarity. The intravasation of a large amount of hypotonic fluid results in a simultaneous drop of serum sodium levels. Ghanem and Ward showed that of the 11 of 100 patients who absorbed greater than 1 L of glycine, 7 developed symptoms of TURP syndrome.[36] The development of symptoms was most strongly linked with a mean total operative volumetric fluid absorption of 3.54 L (glycine and IV solution) in men who weighed 70 kg. These findings suggest that in an average female patient weighing 60 kg, as little as a total absorption of 3 L of fluid can precipitate symptoms of "post-TURP" syndrome.

Initially, if a large volume of hypo-osmotic glycine solution is intravasated, the serum osmolality does not change. Glycine has an intravascular half-life of 85 minutes, and for that period of time helps to maintain serum osmolarity. Serum sodium levels, however, will be lower, and early detection and treatment of hyponatremia within this window of time will obviate any sequelae. After that time period, the intravasated glycine is absorbed intracellularly, and eventually a large surplus of free water is generated from the intravasated distention medium. If untreated, hypo-osmolar hyponatremia results. This process is further accelerated by the release of antidiuretic hormone in response to the stress of surgery. In addition, female patients are thought to be more susceptible to hyponatremia as progesterone has been shown to inhibit the cellular sodium-potassium ATP enzyme.[21,26,38] Finally, the use of vasopressin to thwart intraoperative bleeding will further contribute to the renal absorption of free water and accelerate the development of hypervolemic/hypo-osmolar hyponatremia.

The neurologic complications of hypo-osmotic hypervolemia stem largely from the rapid movement of free water across the blood-brain barrier and into the brain as equilibration takes place. Intracellular fluid volume is increased, the brain expands and swells within its bony confines. Intracranial pressure increases, cerebral blood flow decreases, and neurons become increasingly hypoxemic.[39] As little as a 5% increase in intracranial volume may lead to brain herniation.[39]

Because hypervolemic/hyponatremic encephalopathy can result in death or permanent brain damage, the goal should lie primarily in preventing this disorder, followed by rapid intervention when there is intravasation of large quantities of fluid. No clear standard has been set for the maximum amount of fluid that can safely be absorbed before operative hysteroscopic procedures should be terminated. However, most authors suggest assessment of the patient's status and discontinuation of the procedure at a fluid deficit of approximately 1 to 1.5 L.[8,31,40] Lower limits, such as 750 ml, should be used for older patients or patients with cardiovascular compromise.[8] Patients who are especially at risk for complications are those with pre-existing liver disease or structural lesions of the central nervous system, those who have experienced a hypoxemic event, and those who use diuretics on a chronic basis.

These complications can largely be avoided by limiting the amount of fluid absorbed. Clearly, longer procedure times are associated with the absorption of larger volumes of fluid. Urologists have long supported limiting the TURP procedure time to less than an hour. Most authors report an average procedure length of less than 45 minutes for operative hysteroscopic procedures and an average fluid deficit of less than 300 ml.[30,40] In each of the four cases of severe hyponatremia associated with endometrial ablation reported by Arieff and Ayus,[35] the operative time was greater than 120 minutes. Operative time appears to be uniformly decreased for ablation and resection procedures by pretreatment with danazol (Danocrine), or gonadotropin-releasing hormone (GnRH) agonists.[24,41] Magos et al[24] reported an average procedure time of 40 minutes and an average absorption of fluid of 687 ml for patients who had not been treated with danazol before hysteroscopic myomectomy, compared with less than 20 minutes and 125 ml for patients who had been pretreated.

These findings are further reinforced by Donnez et al,[42] who reported an average overall decrease of 450 ml of intravasated fluid for patients treated with GnRH agonists before hysteroscopic myomectomy, compared with those who were not pretreated. The reduction in fluid absorption was largely attributed to a decrease in uterine cavity size (36%) and a decrease in myoma size (range 4% to 90%, average 38%). Reduced fluid absorption has also been attributed to a decrease in endometrial vascularity. Treatment with GnRH agonists has been shown to decrease blood flow to the uterus.[24] Certainly, pretreatment with danazol or GnRH agonists has been associated with a thinner endometrium and improved surgical outcomes.[42-45]

Once fluid overload is recognized, rapid intervention is of utmost importance. Failure to treat acute (less than 48 hours) hyponatremia with diuresis and hypertonic saline may lead to the development of neurologic symptoms, and progress to a persistent vegetative state or death.[39] Often patients with severe hyponatremia can deteriorate rapidly and without warning. Sterns[46] reported on a series of 15 previously healthy women who underwent elective surgery and subsequently developed severe hyponatremia. In less than 10 minutes and without warning, 8 of 15 alert patients experienced a grand mal seizure followed by respiratory arrest.

Although the rate at which severe hyponatremia should be treated is controversial, most authors agree that if acute hyponatremia has existed for less than 24 hours there are few long-term complications associated with a "rapid" correction. Therapy is most frequently provided in the form of hypertonic sodium chloride (514 mmol/L), in conjunction with a loop-acting diuretic such as furosemide. Serum sodium levels may be safely increased by 1 to 2 mEq/L per hour during the first few hours, with a maximum increase of approximately 12 mEq/L in the first 24 hours.[21,46] However, the following circumstances can lead to permanent brain injury in patients with hyponatremia: (1) increasing the serum sodium concentration by greater than 25 mmol during the initial 48 hours of therapy, (2) overcorrection to hypernatremic levels, and (3) increasing serum sodium from normonatremic to hypernatremic levels in patients with either severe liver disease or other debilitating medical illnesses.[39] The goal of therapy should be to aim for slightly *hyponatremic* serum levels to avoid overcorrection.

Diuresis may also be accomplished with mannitol. Some authors favor this therapy because mannitol is an osmotic diuretic that leads to less sodium loss in the urine.[21] However, mannitol is an effective intravascular osmol and may rapidly increase the intravascular volume further, adding to preload volumes and thereby increasing myocardial oxygen demand. This may pose a problem for patients with borderline cardiovascular function and place them at increased risk for congestive heart failure and myocardial ischemia. For this reason, the use of furosemide has been supported primarily to achieve adequate diuresis. In patients with normal renal function, 20 mg intravenously has been shown to establish adequate diuresis.[21] Larger doses may be required in patients with renal disease. Urine output should be measured accurately with an indwelling foley catheter, and serum electrolytes should be monitored every 2 to 4 hours.

Concern related to correction of severe hyponatremia stems largely from the more chronic (greater than 48 hours) form of the disorder. Rapid correction of hyponatremia in this setting has been said to cause an obscure neurologic disorder called "central pontine myelinolysis" (CPM).[46] Patients with mild symptoms (i.e., weakness, dysarthria, confusion) or severe symptoms (i.e., seizures and coma) of hyponatremia appear to improve initially during correction of the electrolyte disturbance. However, after partial or complete correction, the patient's neurologic condition deteriorates, and new clinical findings emerge. In the fully developed syndrome, the patient develops quadriparesis, mutism, and pseudobulbar palsy.[21,39,46] Seizures, behavioral disturbances, and movement disorders can also be seen.

CPM is thought by some to represent the injury suffered as a result of brain desiccation from too rapid a correction of chronic hyponatremia.[46] In the acute form, the brain is resistant to the influx of free water and is able to shunt fluid into the cerebrospinal fluid (CSF). However, the ability to unload fluid is time-dependent, and dumping free water is then followed by the shunting of sodium and water. In the face of continued hyponatremia, neurons first extrude potassium, followed by a loss of cytoplasmic organic osmolytes (i.e., taurine, myoinositol, glutamine, glutamate, and phosphocreatine).[26] Because the intracellular regeneration of these osmols takes several days, a rapid increase in serum osmolality related to correction results in the further movement of free water out of the neurons, thereby predisposing them to dehydration. This scenario has been the proposed mechanism of CPM, whose pathognomonic lesion is demyelination in all areas of the brain, including the pons.[39] These lesions may be detected on computed tomography (CT) and magnetic resonance imaging (MRI) within 4 weeks of clinical onset.

The exclusive role of rapid correction of "chronic" (greater than 48 hours) hyponatremia as the etiologic factor in CPM is not uniformly held. As stated previously, the lesions are invariably distributed in many other parts of the brain besides the pons.[39] CPM is most common in patients who have liver cirrhosis, have suffered cardiopulmonary arrest or carbon monoxide poisoning, or have untreated hyponatremia. Some authors have proposed hypoxic brain damage as a major influence in the development of this neurologic disorder.[39] Because cerebral hypoxemia is a known complication of untreated severe hyponatremia, it follows that there is a higher preponderance of these demyelination lesions in patients who suffer from these symptoms.

Besides the neurologic complications associated with hyponatremia, several cases of encephalopathy secondary to elevated serum ammonia levels have been reported.[21,47,48] Glycine is a nonessential amino acid that is normally present in the circulation. Oxidative deamination of glycine in the liver and kidneys normally results in the formation of small quantities of glyoxylic acid and ammonia.[5,39] The intravascular absorption of large quantities of glycine could result in a marked increase in the concentration of blood ammonia. Patients vary tremendously in the amount of ammonia they produce in response to elevated serum glycine levels, and patients with liver disease do not appear to be at increased risk for the development of hyperammonemia. Therefore it is not possible to predict which patients are at risk for developing an encephalopathy from the metabolism of glycine. Ammonia toxicity should be suspected in patients who exhibit central nervous system depression following a procedure with glycine in whom the degree of hyponatremia does not explain the full extent of their symptoms.

The use of glycine solutions has been associated with transient blurry vision, and even transient blindness following TURP procedures.[8,21] Under normal circumstances, glycine acts as an inhibitory neurotransmitter in the ganglion and horizontal cells of the retina.[21] Therefore, under circumstances in which the level is transiently increased, visual changes may occur.

Sorbitol and mannitol. Solutions containing 2.7% sorbitol and 0.54% mannitol are commercially available, nonconductive, and have been used for both TURP procedures and for "rollerball" endometrial ablation procedures.[40] Sorbitol and mannitol are six-carbon alditol isomers. Sorbitol is metabolized by the liver to glucose and fructose. Mannitol is primarily cleared by the kidneys and excreted largely unchanged in the urine. Some authors encourage the use of solutions containing mannitol because of its short plasma half-life (15 minutes) and its effect as an osmotic diuretic.[21,49] Theoretically, the use of mannitol should reduce the risk of fluid overload.

Solutions of sorbitol and mannitol, like glycine, are supplied in 3-liter bags. The method of use, the indications for use, and the expected possible complications are similar to glycine.

Normal saline. The use of normal saline has been reported for operative hysteroscopic procedures that do not require electrosurgical techniques. The major advantages associated with it are its availability, its nonrisk of hyponatremia, and the ease of diuresis should volume overload occur. However, as an electrolyte solution, it diffuses and renders the diathermy current ineffective and it cannot be used with the resectoscope.[21] Therefore, normal saline has restricted applications in therapeutic hysteroscopic procedures. It is commonly used during intrauterine laser procedures and procedures using rigid, semirigid, and flexible instruments such as polyp and biopsy forceps or scissors.

CONCLUSION

For diagnostic office hysteroscopy, a panoramic view of the uterine cavity is best achieved with either nonviscous, isotonic solutions such as normal saline infused via a 60-ml syringe and IV tubing or CO_2 infused with a hysteroscopic insufflator. Hyskon should be used only if the procedure is being performed on an emergency basis while the patient is actively bleeding and a clear view cannot otherwise be obtained, and then only with a noncontinuous-flow hysteroscope. Its use for therapeutic procedures is limited to those that can be completed with relatively small volumes of distention media and are of short duration. Glycine and sorbitol/mannitol solutions are well-established hypotonic distending media for use with the continuous-flow resectoscope. There is no place for them, however, if electricity is not being used. Isotonic, nonviscous solutions should be used with the Nd:YAG laser and the operative hysteroscope.

Although the potential complications have been stressed, each medium is safe when used within the confines of specific restrictions. For example, CO_2 must be delivered by an hysteroscopic insufflator, not more than 500 ml of dextran should be used for any one procedure, and the fluid deficit should be monitored closely for hypo-osmolar solutions. GnRH agonists or danazol serve as important adjunctive therapies and can help limit intravasation of distention media. Prevention and attention to detail during the course of hysteroscopic procedures will minimize the chance for complications. Recognition and the early intervention of therapy will minimize the potential for serious sequelae resulting from the intravasation of excessive quantities of distention media.

REFERENCES

1. Lindeman HJ, Mohr J: CO_2 hysteroscopy: diagnosis and treatment, *Am J Obstet Gynecol* 124(2):129-133, 1976.
2. Siegler AM, Kemmann E: Hysteroscopy, *Obstet Gynecol Surv* 30(9):567-588, 1975.
3. Corson SL et al: Cardiopulmonary effects of direct venous CO_2 insufflation in ewes, *J Report Med* 33(5):440-444, 1988.
4. Hulka JF et al: Operative hysteroscopy American Association of Gynecologic Laparoscopists 1991 membership survey, *J Reprod Med,* 38(8), 1993.
5. Baggish MS, Daniell JF: Death caused by air embolism associated with neodymium:yttrium-aluminum-garnet laser surgery and artificial sapphire tips, *Am J Obstet Gynecol* 161:877-878, 1989.
6. Challener RC, Kaufman B: Fatal venous air embolism following sequential unsheathed (bare) and sheathed quartz fiber Nd:YAG laser endometrial ablation, *Anesthesiology* 73:548-551, 1990.
7. Perry PM, Baughman VL: A complication of hysteroscopy: air embolism, *Anesthesiology* 73:546-547, 1990.
8. Brooks PG: Complications of operative hysteroscopy: how safe is it, *Clin Obstet Gynecol* 35(2):256-261, 1992.
9. De Jong P, Doel F, Falconer A: Outpatient diagnostic hysteroscopy, *Br J Obstet Gynaecol* 97:299-303, 1990.
10. Gimpelson RJ: Preventing cervical reflux of the distention medium during panoramic hysteroscopy, *J Reprod Med* 31(7):592-594, 1986.
11. Gomel V et al: *Laparoscopy and hysteroscopy in gynecologic practice,* Chicago, 1986, Year Book Medical Publishers.
12. DeCherney AH et al: Endometrial ablation for intractable uterine bleeding: hysteroscopic resection, *Obstet Gynecol* 70(4):668-670, 1987.
13. Brandt RR, Dunn WF, Ory SJ: Dextran 70 embolization: another cause of pulmonary hemorrhage, coagulopathy, and rhabdomyolysis, *Chest* 104(2):631-633, 1993.
14. Golan A et al: High-output left ventricular failure after dextran use in an operative hysteroscopy, *Fertil Steril* 54(5):939-941, 1990.
15. Leake JF, Murphy AA, Zacur HA: Noncardiogenic pulmonary edema: a complication of operative hysteroscopy, *Fertil Steril* 48(3):497-499, 1987.
16. Manger D et al: Pulmonary edema and coagulopathy due to Hyskon (32% dextran 70) administration, *Anesth Analg* 68:686-687, 1989.
17. Vercellini P et al: Hypervolemic pulmonary edema and severe coagulopathy after intrauterine dextran instillation, *Obstet Gynecol* 79(5):838-839, 1992.
18. Zbella EA, Moise J, Carson SA: Noncardiogenic pulmonary edema secondary to intrauterine instillation of 32% dextran 70, *Fertil Steril* 43(3):479-480.
19. Moran M, Kapsner C: Acute renal failure associated with elevated plasma oncotic pressure, *N Engl J Med* 317(3):150-152, 1987.
20. Lukacsko P: Noncardiogenic pulmonary edema secondary to intrauterine instillation of 32% dextran 70, *Fertil Steril* 44(4):560-561, 1985.
21. Witz CA et al: Complications associated with the absorption of hysteroscopic fluid media, *Fertil Steril* 60(5):745-756, 1993.
22. Kaplan AI, Sabin S: Dextran 40: another cause of drug-induced noncardiogenic pulmonary edema, *Chest* 68(3):376-377, 1975.
23. Jedeikin R, Olsfanger D, Kessler I: Disseminated intravascular coagulopathy and adult respiratory distress syndrome: life-threatening complications of hysteroscopy, *Am J Obstet Gynecol* 162:44-45, 1990.
24. Magos AL et al: Experience with the first 250 endometrial resections for menorrhagia, *Lancet* 377:1074-1078, 1991.
25. Data JL, Nies AS: Dextran 40, *Ann Intern Med* 81:500-504, 1974.
26. Andrew RD: Seizure and acute osmotic change: clinical and neurophysiological aspects, *J Neurol Sci.* 10(1):7-18, 1991.
27. Ahmed N et al: Anaphylactic reaction because of intrauterine 32% dextran 70 instillation, *Fertil Steril* 55(5):1014-1016, 1991.
28. Bailey G et al: Dextran-induced anaphylaxis, *JAMA* 200(10):889-891, 1967.
29. Trimbos-Kemper TCM, Veering BT: Anaphylactic shock from intracavitary 32% dextran 70 during hysteroscopy, *Fertil Steril* 51(60): 1053-1054, 1989.
30. Vulgaropulos SP: Intrauterine pressure and fluid absorption during continuous flow hysteroscopy, *Am J Obstet Gynecol* 167(2):386-387, 1992.
31. Istre O et al: Transcervical resection of endometrium and fibroids: initial complications, *Acta Obstet Gynecol Scand* 70:363-366, 1991.
32. Garry R: Safety of hysteroscopic surgery, *Lancet* 336:1013-1014, 1990.
33. Siegler AM, Valle RF: Therapeutic hysteroscopic procedures, *Fertil Steril* 50(5):685-701, 1988.
34. Schinagl EF: Hyskon (32% dextran 70), Hysteroscopic surgery and pulmonary edema, *Anesth Analg* 70:223-224, 1990.
35. Arieff AI, Ayus J: Endometrial ablation complicated by fatal hyponatremic encephalopathy, *JAMA* 270(10):1230-1232, 1993.
36. Ghanem AN, Ward JP: Osmotic and metabolic sequelae of volumetric overload in relation to the TURP syndrome, *Brit J Urol* 66:71-78, 1990.
37. Hahn RG: Fluid and electrolyte dynamics during development of the TURP syndrome, *Brit J Urol* 66:79-84, 1990.
38. Arieff AI: Hyponatremia, convulsions, respiratory arrest, and permanent brain damage after elective surgery in healthy women, *N Engl J Med* 314(24);1529-1535.
39. Arieff AI: Treatment of symptomatic hyponatremia: Neither haste nor waste, *Crit Care Med* 19(6):748-751, 1991.
40. Townsend DE et al: "Rollerball" coagulation of the endometrium, *Obstet Gynecol* 76(2):310-313, 1990.

41. McLucas B: Intrauterine applications of the resectoscope, *Surg Gynecol Obstet* 172(6):425-431, 1991.

42. Donnez J et al: Neodymium:YAG laser hysteroscopy in large submucous fibroids, *Fertil Steril* 54(6):999-1003, 1990.

43. Goldrath MH: Use of danazol in hysteroscopic surgery for menorrhagia, *J Reprod Med* 35(1):91-96, 1990.

44. Vancaillie TG: Electrocoagulation of the endometrium with the ball-end resectoscope, *Obstet Gynecol* 74(3), 425-427, 1989.

45. Wortman M, Daggett A: Hysteroscopic management of intractable uterine bleeding: a review of 103 cases, *J Reprod Med* 38(7):505-510, 1993.

46. Sterns RH: The treatment of hyponatremia: first, do not harm, *Am J Med* 88:557-560, 1990.

47. Hoekstra PT et al: Transurethral prostatic resection syndrome—a new perspective: encephalopathy with associated hyperammonemia, *J Urol* 130:704-707, 1983.

48. Roesch RP et al: Ammonia toxicity resulting from glycine absorption during a transurethral resection of the prostate, *Anesthesiology* 58:577-579, 1983.

49. Van Boven MJ et al: Dilutional hyponatremia associated with intrauterine endoscopic laser surgery, *Anesthesiology* 71:40-451, 1989.

Chapter 7

TECHNIQUES FOR DIAGNOSTIC RIGID HYSTEROSCOPY

Franklin D. Loffer

Performing diagnostic hysteroscopy in an office setting provides benefits for both the patient and her physician. First, there is a savings in time. Counseling the patient, preparing for and performing the procedure, and discussing the findings take only slightly more time than does an office colposcopy for an abnormal pap smear. The physician also avoids travel time and a wait should a case scheduled earlier in the operating room run late. Secondly, it is convenient. Neither the patient nor the physician needs to complete the forms and other papers that would be required by hospitals and outpatient surgical facilities. Furthermore, because diagnostic hysteroscopy is an office procedure, the patient can be scheduled without delay. Office hysteroscopies can often be done during the same visit as when the patient reports her problem. Finally, office hysteroscopy offers a monetary benefit not only in time and convenience but also in actual costs and charges.

PATIENT SELECTION

Most diagnostic hysteroscopies can be performed in an office setting. The majority is done to evaluate abnormal bleeding. A smaller number are done to evaluate the findings of an abnormal hysterosalpingogram, or as a follow-up to evaluate previous intrauterine surgery such as the removal of fibroids, transection of a septum, or lysis of adhesions.

A review of the past 2 years of my private practice experience has indicated that 110 of 130 diagnostic hysteroscopies (84.6%) were performed in the office. Many of those patients whose hysteroscopies were done in a surgical facility also required a laparoscopic examination. Had only a hysteroscopy been indicated, these patients most likely could have had the procedure done in the office.

Only a few patients are not good candidates for office hysteroscopy. The first group of these include the occasional patients who are so anxious that it is difficult to expose the cervix to do even a pap smear. Although it is not necessary that the abdominal musculature be relaxed to do hysteroscopy, it is necessary for reasonable ease of cervical exposure. The second and larger group of patients who may not tolerate office hysteroscopic examinations are older and/or virginal women who have a stenotic and rigid vaginal canal or whose cervix is flush with the vaginal vault. It is very difficult to gain adequate exposure without causing discomfort in these patients.

The ideal time during the menstrual cycle to accomplish hysteroscopy is immediately after the flow has ceased. Then the endometrium is thin, and small lesions are readily visible. When the procedure is done later in the cycle, secretory endometrium may assume a somewhat polypoid appearance and be thick enough to cover small lesions. In addition, when traumatized, late proliferative and secretory endometrium bleeds more easily, which makes visualization difficult. It is not always possible to schedule patients in the early proliferative period. Some procedures will have to be done during the secretory phase and even during active uterine bleeding. Although this is feasible, it is not desirable unless a 5.5-mm O.D. continuous-flow hysteroscope is available, or Hyskon is used for distention.

COUNSELING THE PATIENT

One of the most important aspects of office hysteroscopy is educating the patient about what to expect. The American College of Obstetricians and Gynecologists published an informational brochure (Hysteroscopy AP 084) that is very helpful. This brochure can be given to the patient in advance of the examination. Before taking the patient to the examination room, explain to her the procedure and what she can expect during it. I prefer to do this in my consultative office. Family members are encouraged to be present for the counseling and, if they wish, the procedure. During counseling, each aspect of the procedure is explained step by step so the patient will understand what to expect. The following list shows the sequence of this discussion and some of the wording I use:

1. Positioning of the patient—"Your legs will be cradled in stirrups."
2. Prepping—"The vaginal area will be washed."
3. Injection of the local anesthetic—"This may not be felt. If it is, it most often is described as a pinching or cramping sensation."
4. Performance of hysteroscopy—"Menstrual-like cramping may or may not occur. This portion of the procedure takes only a matter of several minutes if good visualization is being obtained."
5. Performance of an aspiration curettage—"If tissue needs to be sent to the pathologist, there will be menstrual cramping. This portion of the procedure lasts 30 seconds or less."
6. Discussion of the findings—"We will talk back in the consultative office when we have finished."

PROCEDURE ROOM SETUP

Office hysteroscopy is greatly facilitated by having an equipped procedure room. It is very difficult to successfully perform office hysteroscopy without an appropriate examination table, equipment, and supplies. This room need not be elaborate but should contain the equipment necessary to perform the procedure, as well as to respond to an emergency should one arise. Commercial emergency kits are available, or individual items can be assembled as shown in the box below.

After opening the outer covering of the prepping basin and main instrument tray, the surgeon will use sterile gloves for the remainder of the procedure. The assistant does not

---

Emergency supplies

O_2 tank with nose tongs
Ambu respiration bag
Oral airway
IV pole
IV tubing
IV fluids (D5/RL)
Atropine
Sodium bicarbonate
Epinephrine
Syringes and needles
Tourniquet

---

need to wear sterile gloves. Sterile gowns are not used, but surgeons will need either a smock or a clean disposable gown that can be reused to prevent soiling their clothing.

PATIENT PREPARATION

Thirty to sixty minutes before the procedure, the patient is given a prostaglandin synthesis inhibitor. Administering such a drug not only will decrease the amount of cramping the patient may experience but also will provide some psychologic support that she has been given an "anti-pain" medication. The patient is allowed to empty her bladder, more for her comfort than to facilitate the procedure. Her blood pressure, pulse, and a recent weight are recorded as a baseline. The lower portion of her clothing is removed, and her lower abdomen and legs are draped. She then is asked to lie back, and her legs are comfortably positioned in the stirrups. The patient must not be required to actively support her legs during the procedure. It is important that she be able to relax her legs and thus her pelvic musculature. Her buttocks should be at the end of the table. Care is taken that any of the clothing she is still wearing is well away from the buttocks to avoid its being soiled with the prepping solution or from any bleeding that might occur.

A small prepping basin is then opened on the shelf beneath the perineum. The sponges are soaked by the assistant with povidone-iodine or a similar cleansing solution. The sponges are held by a ring forceps, which has been taken from the main tray that sits next to the hysteroscopist. While the vulva and vagina are being cleansed, the hysteroscopist should acknowledge to the patient that this step is not a pleasant one. Expressing this will help reassure the patient that the hysteroscopist is sensitive to her discomfort.

When the cervix is exposed for cleansing, the patient is told that a speculum "just like we use for all routine examinations" will be inserted. This speculum should be one-sided in case it must be removed after the hysteroscope has been inserted. Removing the speculum may be necessary to allow manipulation of the telescope in an acutely anteflexed or retroflexed uterus. During cleansing of the cervix, an effort is made to wash away any cervical mucus.

The prepping bowl and its cover, which has functioned as a temporary sterile field, is removed, and another sterile pad is placed beneath the patient's buttocks and over the perineal tray. No other draping is used.

Although it is my preference to use povidone-iodine or a similar agent as a prepping solution, some hysteroscopists believe that prepping is unnecessary because the vagina cannot be sterilized.

ANESTHESIA

In most cases, it is possible to insert a rigid 5-mm diagnostic hysteroscopic sheath or a flexible hysteroscope into the uterine cavity and obtain adequate visualization without using an anesthetic agent. These instruments are essentially the same size as many intrauterine devices, which generally do not require cervical dilatation. Distention of the cavity at the pressures required for office hysteroscopy is not particularly uncomfortable. Contact with the uterine wall at the time tissue is taken for biopsy or aspiration curettage causes more discomfort. In more than 95% of cases in which only diagnostic hysteroscopy is being performed with a 3.6-mm flexible hysteroscope, the surgeon does not need to dilate the cervix or use anesthesia. Because most patients undergoing diagnostic hysteroscopy with rigid instrumentation require some intrauterine manipulation, I prefer to do a paracervical and intracervical block before introducing the hysteroscope.

The cervix has already been exposed for cleansing. I use 10 ml of a 1% lidocaine hydrochloride solution without epinephrine. Other local anesthetic agents can be used. A finger-grip controlled 10-ml syringe with a 3-inch needle extender and a 20-gauge disposable needle is ideal for administering the anesthesia. A 20-gauge spinal needle can also be used. The spinal needle has the advantage of containing less volume from the needle tip to the syringe, and therefore it is easier to demonstrate the intravasculature position of the needle tip on aspiration. However, it is less rigid and tends to bend on insertion.

The needle is first placed into the posterior lip of the cervix, and several milliliters of the anesthetic agent are injected. Before this step, the patient is told that she may experience some pinching or cramping at the time of the injection. After the anesthetic has been injected, the posterior lip of the cervix is grasped with a tenaculum and raised anteriorly to help delineate the uterosacral ligaments. As this is done, the patient is told that she will feel some manipulation (of the cervix) and maybe some pressure or cramping. Several milliliters of lidocaine hydrochloride are then injected immediately below the vaginal mucosa over each uterosacral ligament. The ligament itself is not injected. The intracervical block is then done. Although some clinicians inject the anesthetic into the cervical stroma, I find this exceedingly difficult. Instead, I inject several more milliliters beneath the cervical mucosa at approximately 9, 12, and 3 o'clock. Usually a small amount of lidocaine hydrochloride remains in the syringe. This is then injected between the uterosacrals at their junction with the cervix. The tenaculum is then moved to the anterior lip of the cervix. Although bleeding frequently occurs at the site where the posterior cervical lip was injected, it has no significance and will stop spontaneously. Now the patient is told that the administration of anesthetic has been completed, and a sponge is being placed in the vagina to tamponade and absorb any bleeding that might occur. The anesthetic may take up to 10 minutes to become fully effective. During this time, the hysteroscopist can rinse, dry, and assemble the hysteroscopic equipment being used. While this is being done, the assistant and hysteroscopist should make an effort to talk to the patient about unrelated matters and reassure her that she will be notified in advance of any further activity involving her.

PREPARING THE OPERATIVE FIELD

Preparation for anesthesia consisted of opening the prepping basin in front of the patient's perineum and using the covering sheet as a temporary drape. After this sheet is removed, another drape is slipped beneath the patient's buttocks. This drape is small (24 inches square) and just large enough to overlap the tray.

Before injecting the anesthetic, the hysteroscopist opens the tray containing the equipment, which has been autoclaved. The telescope and fiberoptic cable, which have been soaked, are now taken from the disinfection solution, dried, and assembled with the sheath. When the equipment has been assembled and is ready for use, the light source and CO_2 insufflator are turned on. The patient is forewarned about the fan noise made by the light source.

A convenient way to drape the light and distending medium tubing onto the platform covered with the sterile drape is to clip a sterile hemostat to the drape covering the stirrup. The cables are then passed through and supported by the finger grips of the hemostat.

INSERTION OF THE HYSTEROSCOPE

When the operative field has been prepared and the hysteroscope is ready for introduction, the patient is told she will feel the sponge being removed from the vagina. It is often quite bloody, and the vagina may need to be sponged again with a dry 4×4 gauze pad. An effort is made to remove any mucus that may remain at the cervical opening. If CO_2 is being used for uterine distention, mucus that is pushed ahead of the telescope will hinder good visualization. Some physicians introduce the rigid hysteroscope without using a tenaculum to stabilize the cervix. Although this is feasible, it has always been my preference to straighten the cervical-uterine axis by downward traction of the tenaculum, which is attached to the anterior cervical lip. When using the flexible hysteroscope, a tenaculum is generally not necessary because the scope can be manipulated through the curved cervical canal.

Dilatation of the cervix is seldom necessary and should be done only when the need is demonstrated. It usually is not necessary even in postmenopausal patients in whom the cervical os appears quite small. In these patients, the canal is usually of adequate diameter. The apparent narrowness is simply the growth of the cervical epithelium over the os. Occasionally, if there is difficulty in introducing the telescope, it may be necessary to use a small cervical dilator. Under such circumstances, only the external os needs to be dilated. It is necessary to dilate the cervix only to the diameter of the scope to be introduced (3.6 to 5.5 mm).

When the telescope is inserted, the patient is told that she will feel some motion and possibly some menstrual-like cramping. The scope should be inserted under direct vision. Particular attention should be given to the view obtained by a rigid foreoblique scope. The angles of view of all foreoblique scopes vary between 12° and 30° off the axis of the scope. This means that when the scope is placed directly down the cervical canal, and the angle of vision is anterior, the roof of the canal will be seen and the apparent opening of the cervix is in the 6 o'clock position. This relationship will change depending on the direction in which the scope is rotated. When the cervical canal appears in the middle of the field of vision, the scope is being directed into the wall of the cervical canal, which will cause pain and bleeding and prevent advancement of the scope (Fig. 7-1). This situation does not apply to

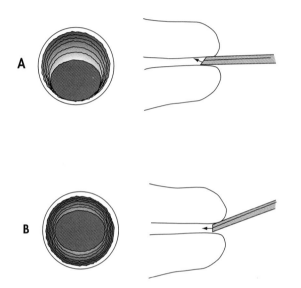

Fig. 7-1. Correct vs. incorrect entry of the hysteroscope. **A,** When a hysteroscope with a foreoblique view is inserted into the cervix, the cervical canal should appear below the tip of the scope. **B,** If the canal appears in the center of the view, the scope is being inserted incorrectly. (Reproduced with permission from Loffer FD: Ambulatory obstetrical and gynecological surgery. In Davis JE, Ed: *Major ambulatory surgery,* Baltimore, 1986, Williams & Wilkins.)

flexible hysteroscopes, which have a 0° angle of view. In these scopes, the view seen is the actual one (See Chapter 8.)

Usually the cervical canal will open widely, and the direction of passage easily noted. When this does not occur, the hysteroscopist should look for movement of the distending medium to indicate the location of the canal and the area to which the scope should be directed. When CO_2 is used, it is possible to follow the progression of the medium, which appears as small bubbles moving into the uterine cavity. When fluid is used, the actual flow of the medium can be identified.

When CO_2 is used, the flow rate should be no more than 50 cc a minute with a maximum pressure of 100 mg Hg. If fluids are used, pressure via the plunger on a syringe or via a blood pressure cuff should be adjusted to allow for adequate fluid flow and uterine distention. In general, 75 mm Hg is sufficient for adequate visualization but this is not routinely measured during office hysteroscopy, and isotonic fluid intravasation is not a significant risk in short diagnostic cases.[1] Higher pressures are uncomfortable for the patient, and the assistant should relax on the syringe until the patient is comfortable.

The scope should not be introduced rapidly because this will create discomfort and bubbles if CO_2 is being used. Also the hysteroscope should always be inserted under direct vision. However, on occasion the uterus is very anteflexed or retroflexed, and the direction of the canal can be seen but the beveled end of the rigid scope prevents easy introduction. When this occurs, it is not necessary to dilate the cervix. The scope can simply be kept in the same axis but rotated 180°.

While direct visualization is lost, the beveled edge acts as a sled to allow the scope to be inserted into the uterine cavity (Fig. 7-2).

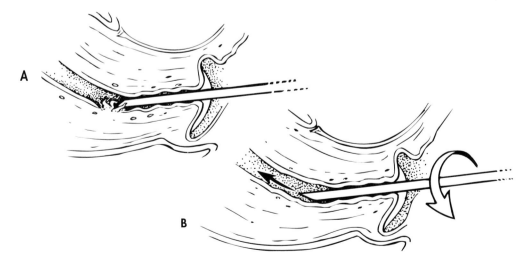

Fig. 7-2. Transversing an angled cervical canal. **A,** Further insertion is blocked. **B,** Insertion is facilitated by rotation of a beveled end of the telescope. (Reproduced with permission from Loffer FD: Hysteroscopy. In Stangel JJ, Ed: *Infertility surgery: a multimethod approach to female reproductive surgery,* New York, 1990, Appleton & Lange.)

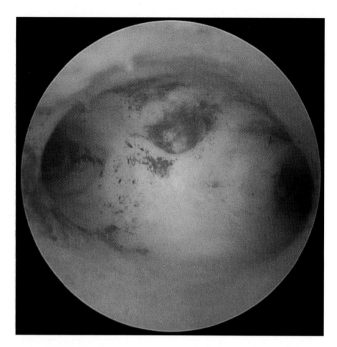

Fig. 7-3. An overall view of the uterine cavity. This is accomplished by bringing the hysteroscope into the upper cervical canal.

VISUALIZATION OF THE CAVITY

Theoretically, the cervical canal, lower uterine segment, and fundus are visualized in that order as the hysteroscope is introduced. From a practical point, the canal is best visualized as the hysteroscope is withdrawn at the end of the diagnostic procedure. To best visualize the uterine cavity, the hysteroscopist inserts the hysteroscope into the uterine cavity to the fundus and then withdraws it into the junction of the lower uterine segment and upper cervical canal. This maneuver is very important because it is from this point that the entire uterine cavity can be visualized (Fig. 7-3).

The hysteroscopist should see the typical slightly arcuate shape of the uterine cavity and the tubal ostia located in each horn. If this view is not obtained, the hysteroscopist must make an effort to find out why. There may be an abnormality such as a septum, polyp, fibroid, or tissue preventing an overall view of the cavity. Alternatively, the hysteroscope may not even be in the uterine cavity.

Once an overview of the uterine cavity has been obtained, it is then possible to examine any area in question at closer range by inserting the scope farther into the fundus. When using a riding hysteroscope, the operator should learn to use the foreoblique lenses. Simply rotating the scope on its axis will allow better visualization of each side of the cavity. The direction in which the foreoblique scope is viewing will always have a consistent relationship with the light post on the scope.

As described in Chapter 3, the flexible hysteroscope can scan the cavity by movement of its tip. Although this feature allows even greater maneuverability to view the uterine cavity, it may initially be confusing to the novice hysteroscopist.

OBTAINING A CLEAR VIEW OF THE UTERINE CAVITY

Probably the single most common problem gynecologists have when introducing hysteroscopy into an office setting is obtaining adequate visualization of the uterine cavity. Although this difficulty initially is a source of considerable frustration, it should not be a lasting problem once the techniques and the tricks to obtain good visualization have been mastered (Table 7-1). The most common problem when using CO_2 is the creation of bubbles. These are best prevented by inserting the scope slowly, using a flow rate of less than 50 cc/minute. Quick insertion of the hysteroscope and higher flow rates will churn any mucus and blood that are present and create a frothy view that is difficult to clear. Even when slow insertion and flow rates are used, bubbles may be present in the uterine cavity. The hysteroscopist should initially wait to see if the bubbles clear either by the pressure of the CO_2 expelling them through the fallopian tubes or independently through the canal back alongside the instrument. Occasionally, it will be necessary to shut off the inflow of CO_2 and let the uterus contract. Then, when the valve is reopened, distention may occur without the presence of bubbles. Another technique for decompressing the uterus is to disconnect the CO_2 tubing. This method is more rapid but may allow some of the blood and debris to enter the sheath and simply re-create the problem when the gas is reattached.

Another alternative is to disconnect the CO_2 tubing and inject 20 ml of sterile saline down the inflow channel. The saline will wash the uterine cavity, and the fluids used can be drained back through the sheath and removed with the injecting syringe. The CO_2 is then reattached. Once this is done, better visualization is generally attained. However, some fluid may remain in the uterine cavity, possibly obscuring small lesions on the posterior uterine wall.

Until recently, the most common distending medium for office hysteroscopy has been CO_2. It provides excellent visualization, and is clean and readily suitable for office use. Because bubbles and bleeding can be a problem, however, some hysteroscopists prefer to use Hyskon. It is difficult, however, to inject undiluted Hyskon through a 5-mm rigid diagnostic sheath. Furthermore, although blood is not miscible with Hyskon, it certainly can mix with it, and good visualization is not a guarantee. Recently, continuous-flow diagnostic hysteroscopes suitable for office use have been developed. Although the low-viscosity fluid makes collection and disposal of the distending medium more difficult, the volumes used are small enough not to be a significant problem. Self-contained office systems are available (Circon ACMI, Stamford, Conn.; Olympus America Corp, New York). The use of a continuous-flow system is ideal when good visualization of the cavity is obscured by bubbles, blood, or debris.

Table 7-1. Trouble-shooting reasons for poor visualization of the uterine cavity

Problem	Finding/cause	Diagnosis/solution
No uterine distention	Insufflator indicates high pressure	Check CO_2 tank or cartridge to be sure it is full or on
		Check tightness of connections of tubing or hysteroscope
		Lax cervix: torque or move tenaculum
	Insufflator indicates low pressure	Valve closed
		Telescope against fundus
		Tubing twisted
Difficulty inserting	Insertion angle incorrect	See Fig. 7-1
telescope	Severely anteflexed	
	or retroflexed uterus	See Fig. 7-2
	Stenotic canal	Dilate
	Already at fundus	Stop advancing hysteroscope
Image red	No uterine distention	See above
	Hysteroscope at uterine fundus	Pull back hysteroscope
	Blood on scope	Wipe against fundus
		Remove from sheath and wipe lens
Bubbles	Hysteroscope introduced too quickly	Wait
	or flow rate (CO_2) too high	
		Shut off inflow of CO_2: allow uterine cavity to slowly collapse and redistend
		Disconnect tubing to allow uterine cavity to quickly collapse and immediately reattach
		Inject 10-20 ml sterile saline and let it drain out
		Slowly move hysteroscope around cavity
Uterine cavity filled with	Recent bleeding of thick	Suction curette cavity
blood/tissue	endometrium or tumor	

Occasionally, bubbles are not the problem in obtaining good visualization. Visual obscurity may be secondary either to mucus or a small amount of blood on the lens of the hysteroscope. Under these circumstances, the hysteroscope can be placed against the uterine fundus and gently wiped to clear the view.

Even after trying these techniques, occasionally it will not be possible to get a panoramic view of the uterus. Under these circumstances, it becomes necessary to clear one side of the uterine cavity to determine if abnormalities exist. The other side of the cavity is then cleared, and a view is obtained and combined with the retained mental image of the first side.

It is common to find a clot, a large amount of tissue, or enough free blood in the uterus to obscure the view. In these situations, the hysteroscope can be removed and an aspiration curettage done to remove the blood, clot, or tissue. If the hysteroscope is immediately reinserted, adequate visualization can usually be obtained even when CO_2 is the distending medium. Hyskon and the continuous-flow system may also be used under these circumstances.

Sometimes visualization is not adequate because the uterus is inadequately distended. CO_2 has a low viscosity and can easily leak around the hysteroscope. This problem can be diagnosed by observing a low pressure on the insufflating machine. It can be corrected by torquing the tenaculum, which will tend to tighten the cervix onto the hysteroscope. If this does not work, the tenaculum can be reapplied to the cervix to include more cervical stroma. The external cervical os is then pulled more tightly around the hystero-

scope. Very occasionally, it may be necessary to put a second tenaculum on the posterior aspect of the cervical canal. CO_2 may also be lost if the connections between the scope and the sheath are not tight or if an instrument is placed in the operative channel, with a gasket that does not fit tightly around it. Problems of distention are less common with low-viscosity fluid and virtually nonexistent when high-viscosity Hyskon is used.

SAMPLING THE ENDOMETRIAL TISSUE

The majority of office hysteroscopies will be done to evaluate abnormal bleeding, and therefore tissue sampling will be needed (see Chapter 10). Hysteroscopy with endometrial sampling is a more accurate method of evaluating the causes of abnormal uterine bleeding than are blind procedures such as endometrial biopsy and dilatation and curettage.[2] The primary value of hysteroscopy is to identify polyps and fibroids, which are usually missed by blind procedures; in addition, small areas of abnormal endometrium may be discovered that need to be sent, in addition to the curettage specimen, to the pathologist. Many patients will have a normal uterine cavity and therefore no suspicious areas from which tissue samples need be taken for biopsy.[2] Under these circumstances, the diagnostic hysteroscope may be removed and a blind biopsy specimen obtained by Pipelle suction curettage. Although no further dilatation is necessary, the pressure against the uterine wall causes more discomfort than occurred with the hysteroscopy. The patient should be forewarned about the discomfort she may experience and be told that this part of the procedure will take less time than did the diagnostic hysteroscopy.

Occasionally a small, isolated lesion may be identified. When this occurs, the diagnostic hysteroscope is removed, and a 7-mm operative hysteroscope is inserted. The cervix is frequently relaxed enough that dilatation is not necessary. Although this may cause some increased discomfort, the use of an operative hysteroscope is quite feasible.[3,4] When it is necessary to dilate the cervix, it should be done to a number 14 Hanks dilator (approximately 4.6 mm).

The usual instrument used to obtain a tissue sample for biopsy is a grasping forceps. Most endometrial tissue is soft enough that it can be pulled away from the uterine wall. The tissue is usually not so firmly attached that a biopsy forceps is needed. When a flexible scope is used, the instruments can be introduced directly down the operative channel.

After a specimen of a small lesion has been obtained for biopsy, the cavity is suction-curetted with the same technique as used in the absence of lesions. This step is taken in an effort to send larger amounts of tissue to the pathologist.

CONCLUSION

The purpose of office hysteroscopy is to provide a faster and more accurate diagnosis for both the patient and her physician. It is easily implemented into any gynecologic practice.

REFERENCES

1. Loffer FD: Complications from uterine distension during hysteroscopy. In Corfman RS, Diamond MP, DeCherney A Eds: *Complications of laparoscopy and hysteroscopy,* Cambridge, 1993, Blackwell Scientific Publications.
2. Loffer FD: Hysteroscopy with selective endometrial sampling compared with D&C for abnormal uterine bleeding: the value of a negative hysteroscopic view, *Obstet Gynecol* 73(1):16-20, 1989.
3. Loffer FD: Hysteroscopic sterilization with the use of formed-in-place silicone plugs, *Am J Obstet Gynecol* 149:261-7, 1984.
4. Loffer FD, Loffer PS: Hysteroscopic tubal occlusion with the use of formed-in-place silicone devices: a long-term follow-up, *Gynecol Endoscopy* 1:203-5, 1992.

Chapter 8

NINE YEARS OF EXPERIENCE WITH FLEXIBLE HYSTEROSCOPY

René Marty
Patricia Mussuto

STARTING OUT

Nine years ago, most of our hysteroscopic procedures were conducted under general or local anesthesia. As we became more experienced, we began to schedule patients using only a local anesthetic, but most of the time the procedure was done in a room near the operating room. Eventually we were able to practice office diagnostic fiberhysteroscopy without needing to dilate the cervix in about 90% of cases. The remaining 10% of cases consisted chiefly of postmenopausal women and patients who had had cervical surgery such as conization or laser therapy.

We shall point out our specific technique, which differentiates flexible from rigid hysteroscopy. The following guidelines must be observed to most efficiently use the flexible technique. The procedure generally does not require the use of a tenaculum on the cervix or a preoperative sedative. The adjusting triangular mark in the eyepiece of the hysteroscope must be placed at 0° before the onset of the procedure so that the operator knows where the tip is oriented.

Step 1

When CO_2 or normal saline is infused, the 3.5-mm tip of the hysteroscope is introduced through the external cervical os; then the tip is pushed slowly forward through the cervical canal and advanced smoothly up to the internal os. It is impossible to create a false route. An inexperienced hysteroscopist will not be confused by the true transaxial view obtained with a fiberscope, unlike the rigid instrument, which, with its 12° or 30° foreoblique view, creates an optical illusion.

Progression is made by snaking the hysteroscope through the cervix. The operator must keep the hysteroscope in the center of the cervical canal without touching the walls of the cervix. There is no risk of damage to the cervix, unlike that present with the rigid scope, which has a sharp tip.

Step 2

When the tip has passed the internal cervical os, the entire cavity can be properly visualized with an up-and-down movement of the thumb and/or gentle rotation of the wrist. The best focal length is 2.7 mm. As with any hysteroscopy, after obtaining a general view of the cavity, the gynecologist should observe the endometrial aspect. Then it is time to perform any necessary directed biopsies.

Step 3

The third step is withdrawal of the fiberscope. The device must be withdrawn slowly out of the uterus so that observation of the isthmus and cervical canal can be completed and any pathology missed during the initial insertion can be detected.

By the time the procedure is finished, the quantity of normal saline used for uterine distention usually amounts to no more than 75 to 100 ml.

The average duration of the hysteroscopy ranges from 1 to 12 minutes depending on whether endometrial biopsies are done.

The results of a postoperative pain rating study of 387 patients showed minimal discomfort in 34.4%, some discomfort but easily bearable in 22.2%, and tolerable discomfort equivalent to menstrual cramps in 27.4%.[1]

Patients leave the office about 15 minutes after the end of the procedure, enough time having been allowed to fill the hysteroscopic chart and have a short, final discussion with them.

SPECIAL CASES

Postmenopausal patients

It is sometimes very useful to prepare postmenopausal patients with vaginal estrogen therapy 1 or 2 weeks before hysteroscopy. This treatment softens the atrophic cervix and facilitates insertion of the fiberscope.

Postcervical surgery

Patients who have had cervical surgery, such as cryotherapy, electrotherapy, laser therapy, or conization require a careful evaluation of the external cervical os and sounding of the first centimeter of the cervical canal with a small plastic or rubber probe.

Hysteroscopic procedures during spotting or moderate metrorrhagia

We suggest choosing normal saline rather than CO_2 for distention when the patient is either spotting or experiencing moderate metrorrhagia. This irrigation facilitates the view, clears the clots, and avoids a dirty lens obstructing the view.

Evaluating hormone replacement therapy

If a patient is receiving cyclic hormone replacement therapy, choose the first part of the cycle to perform the procedure to avoid a thick endometrium.

Cervical stenosis

In our practice the rate of cervical stenosis is about 5%. If the cervix must be dilated, the advantage of using a flexible hysteroscope is that we need to dilate only up to 3.5 mm, thereby minimizing the risk of cervical trauma or bleeding. If the patient is too uncomfortable to allow completion of the procedure, *Laminaria* may be used to overcome this difficulty.

VIDEO SETTING

For all our procedures we use a light-sensitive video camera with a xenon light source. This is not a necessity, but, apart from the well-known advantages of the video camera for documentation with a video recorder, we have found that viewing the procedure on a video monitor greatly helps to focus the patient's attention and facilitates the undertaking.

Another advantage is that the video image compares favorably with that of a rigid scope because the quality of the fiber optics has improved dramatically in recent years.

UNDERSTANDING DIAGNOSTIC HYSTEROSCOPIC FINDINGS

Normal hysteroscopic anatomy

The endocervix, which is explored first, is pinkish-yellow. In the nulliparous woman, arborescent folds of the cervical canal stand out while in the multiparous woman they disappear, leaving a flat and smooth endocervix. The internal orifice of the cervix is generally more off-centered compared

with the outer orifice. Therefore, when a rigid endoscope is used, there is a higher risk of perforation if the anatomic curvature is not sufficiently reduced. Once the isthmus is cleared, the cavity takes either a triangular shape, in which the tubal orifices are visible from the internal ostium, or a more tapered shape, in which only the lower uterine segment can be identified from the internal cervical ostium.

During visualization of the tubal orifices, it sometimes is possible to distinguish the intermittent opening and closing of the ostium, attesting to tubal patency. These orifices may be encircled by a yellowish ring, which, according to Parent et al,[2] indicates a *pretubal sphincter* (a barrier between the tubal orifice and the endometrium).

The visual appearance of the endometrium changes according to the phase of the menstrual cycle. In the proliferative phase, the epithelium is thin, has little vascularization, and is yellowish. As the secretory phase approaches, the endometrium thickens and takes on a fluffy aspect with an increasingly pronounced reddish coloration. During this phase, physicians need a lot of eye practice with the flexible hysteroscope to avoid a false diagnosis of hyperplasia and endometrial polyps.

During menopause, the endometrium degenerates, losing its contours and folds, and vascularization becomes rare.

Pathologic hysteroscopic anatomy

One of the more difficult problems in office hysteroscopy is discerning the histologic makeup of lesions that appear grossly similar. For example, submucous myomata seen in the late proliferative phase or secretory phase will often look very similar to endometrial polyps, and endometrial polyps will often resemble polypoid endometrial cancer. Histologic tissue confirmation by direct biopsy is imperative in these circumstances.[2]

Uterine fibroids

Uterine fibroids affect 20% of women over age 35. They are most often detected between the ages of 40 and 50. In 30% of cases, they can be observed at age 20.

The cavity of a uterus with multiple myomata is more difficult to distend with CO_2 than with a liquid medium. However, the intrauterine pressure must still be raised for adequate distention. Submucous fibromas are usually a yellowish-white hemispheric protuberance with a light reflection. Their shape is not altered by the flow of the distention fluid, which attests to their firm consistency (Fig. 8-1). The endometrial thickness covering the myoma is variable and can range from atrophic to hyperplastic. From a few millimeters away, the hysteroscope can trace the surface vascularization over the route of the fibroid's arborescences. Fibromas are sometimes sessile with a large base. When they are on a pedicle, they produce fibrous polyps that can be brought forth through the cervix.

Interstitial myomata are diagnosed by indirect signs, such as the presence of a deformed, cylindric cavity that does not

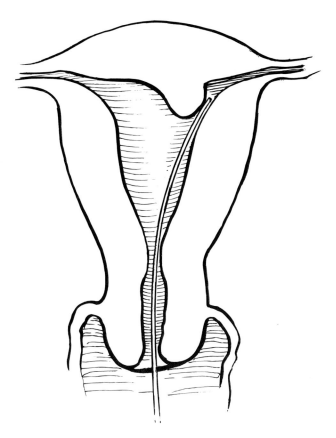

Fig. 8-1. Sessile myoma of uterine bottom.

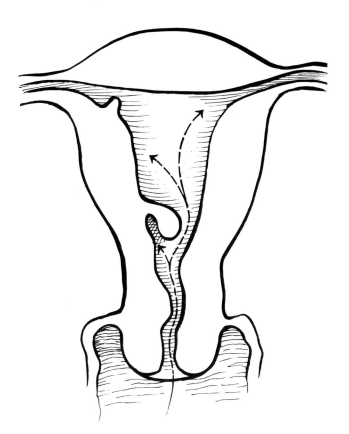

Fig. 8-2. Polymyomatosis and polyps.

permit a panoramic view from the lower uterine segment. They can complicate orientation within the uterine cavity by creating a convex rather than a concave uterine wall, as well as an altered intertubal distance. Their unequal distribution in the myometrium can impede maneuverability within the uterine cavity; therefore, it is important to adapt to these curvatures by using the distal deflective capabilities of the hysteroscope.

Subserous fibromas will go undetected at the hysteroscopic examination.

Whether they are interstitial, submucous, or subserous, 96% of uterine fibroids are found in the uterine corpus whereas only 1% to 3% are found in the cervix. The cervical fibroids are of two types: pedunculated fibromas present in the cervical canal and fibromas within the connective tissue of the endocervix.

Uterine polyps

According to Peterson and Novak,[4] uterine polyps are diagnosed in 60% of premenopausal women, 18% of perimenopausal women, and 28% of postmenopausal women undergoing hysteroscopy.

Functional polyps. *Functional polyps* are also called mucous polyps and represent 36% of all such outgrowths. They are found in women of childbearing age. Their superficial epithelium is glandular and evolves in the same way as normal endometrium. They are quite small, with a 2- to 5-mm diameter, and can have a long pedicle. Their shape varies greatly: they can be hemispheric, conical, or triangular. Their coloring corresponds to that of the nearby endometrium and thus is dependent on the date of the menstrual cycle. The differential diagnosis between a fibroma and a functional polyp is not always easy to make.

Nonfunctional polyps. *Nonfunctional polyps* are more common than functional polyps. Their frequency increases between ages 35 and 50. They are often responsible for metrorrhagia. They vary in size, and their shape is round or oval and more regular than that of functional polyps. Their consistency is halfway between that of a mucous polyp and a fibroma. Because of a thicker superficial endometrial surface, vascularization is less well-detected. Some polyps take up the entire endometrial cavity, obliterating the face of the uterine wall (Fig. 8-2).

Intermediate between the polyp and the myoma is the *adenomyotic polyp.* These outgrowths occur infrequently after menopause. They appear as an undulating and irregular polylobed mass.

In 25% of cases, we have observed the presence of multiple polyps, and in 40% of cases there is a bilesional association of polyps and fibromas.

Degenerated polyps. *Degenerated polyps* are a rare phenomenon. These growths are described as having a

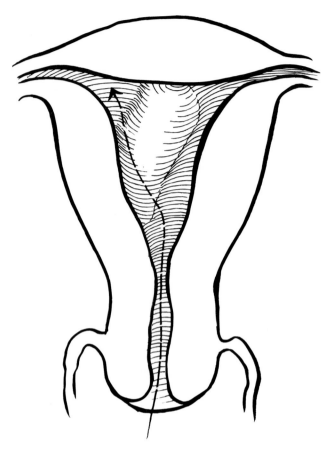

Fig. 8-3. Corporeal synechiae.

healthy base implanted on normal endometrium but with a surface that is a reshaped, eroded mass.

Examination. Every polyp must be examined on all sides, and its entire surface must be explored carefully. If the gynecologist looks only at a polyp's base (or implantation), it is possible to conclude that it is a usual polyp and overlook a suspicious area. The pathologist, however, makes the final diagnosis. In addition, it is necessary to look for polyps in the peritubal areas and under any myoma.

Uterine synechiae

The clinical implications of uterine synechiae vary according to their topography, scope, and duration.

Thin, small, fibrous synechiae can actually be obliterated during hysteroscopy in which a distention medium is used to achieve intracavitary dilatation.

Intrauterine synechiae become a sure obstacle to any rigid hysteroscope when they are isthmic and partially obstruct the lower orifice of the cervical canal. This fibrous reshaping remains difficult to extend despite dilation (Fig. 8-3).

Synechiae do not always have the same physical composition, which can influence the hysteroscopic procedure. Some old synechiae are made of a connective tissue comprising a mixture of collagen and muscular fibers and are similar in appearance to the neighboring endometrium.

Others are purely conjunctival, not very receptive to hormonal impregnation, and characterized by a white, lightly vascularized surface that is smoother than the nearby endometrium.

Marginal synechiae. Marginal synechiae are crescent-shaped lesions composed of a network of multiple whitish and homogenous fibers. They can be oriented in an anterior-posterior, transverse, or oblique direction and can block or reduce access to the tubal orifices.

Endometrial hyperplasia

The generic term *endometrial hyperplasia* refers to quite different anatomic-pathologic varieties, with a specific prognosis for each.[5] However, from an endoscopic point of view, this nuance cannot always be detected. Hysteroscopists must acquire experience to avoid falling into traps such as ignoring well-differentiated local hyperplasia that simulates an isolated, pedunculated polyp.

The endometrium is often divided into blocks that correspond to areas where menstrual desquamation has been incomplete. Examination of the uterine walls in this instance must be thorough so as not to overlook an endometrial tumor.

In the second part of the cycle, it is possible to mistake diffuse hyperplasia for normal secretory endometrium. Examining the tubal orifices can be helpful in distinguishing the two. Except for periods of hemorrhage, the thin, normal endometrium is white. During a heavy period, the intracavitary endometrial shavings become overwhelming, and the coating darkens to a blackish-red shade. The vascularization is dense, but the network remains thin without too many varicosities, unlike that in an endometrial adenocarcinoma.

Adenomyosis

Until recently, adenomyosis could be diagnosed only via hysterectomy. Currently, 80% of uteri with adenomyosis can be detected via MRI. Adenomyosis may be suspected by hysterography when it appears as small channels disseminating from the endometrium into the myometrium. The diagnosis of an interstitial component cannot be made by hysterography. In addition, adenomyosis should be considered when the presence of small bluish or brownish spots impart a punctuate appearance to the endometrial cavity. Even if these hysteroscopic findings suggest adenomyosis, the diagnosis still depends on pathologic interpretation. Currently, the presence of adenomyosis cannot be absolutely confirmed by hysteroscopy.

Endometrial carcinoma

The anatomic-pathologic forms of endometrial carcinoma are varied. The endoscopic appearance must be appraised differently according to whether the distention medium used is physiologic salt solution or CO_2.[6]

Polypoid adenocarcinoma appears as a well-differentiated tubular or glandular lesion. It can also take the shape of a basal polyp but with an irregular surface in some areas. The vascularization is abnormally developed, giving the impression of capillaries meandering here and there.

Nodular carcinoma appears as irregular, knotted projections with a large implantation on the uterine wall. These projections are relatively well-delimited from the neighboring endometrium. They may contain large varicosities that are visible under the surface epithelium.

Papillary adenocarcinoma differs from nodular and polypoid adenocarcinoma by the additional presence of numerous tentacles that float in the liquid medium and cover the projections. Ulcerated adenocarcinoma is the undifferentiated form of endometrial carcinoma. It often appears as a dark, irregular ulceration. The ulcerated carcinoma often contains an underlying infection and is characterized by the presence of pus and necrotic debris. The subepithelial vessels are voluminous and twisting, and in the absence of recent hemorrhage, the color is grayish.

When CO_2 is the distending medium, the appearance of these lesions changes. The pressure of the gas flattens the tentacles associated with the papillary shape and partly erases some malignant projections. In these conditions, the most common presentation is that of a polyped, irregular mass that is widely implanted and distinguishable from healthy tissue. The coloring of the lesion in a gas medium is bluish-white.

The appearance of adenocarcinomas that invade the entire cavity with their irregular and whitish vegetations can be described as "brainlike."

Congenital uterine malformations

Hysterography and laparoscopy remain the gold standard to distinguish between a bicornuate and a septate uterus. However, the flexible hysteroscope can help achieve a precise diagnosis in some difficult clinical cases (Fig. 8-4). A septate uterus will often allow a complete view of the tubal orifices from the level of the internal os. In a bicornuate uterus, visualizing the horns requires progressing the hysteroscope into spaces that are sometimes deeper and narrower than normal. The main value of the flexible hysteroscope, however, is in its therapeutic use with laser resection of uterine septa.

Intrauterine devices

Some IUD removals cannot be performed in an ambulatory setting, and hysteroscopy is indicated to determine the cause. A close-up investigation of the uterine walls may reveal a possible tear or perforation of the uterus, as well as inflammation linked to the presence of a foreign body. The examination evaluates the whole device, as well as its depth of embedment through the endometrium.

THERAPEUTIC OFFICE HYSTEROSCOPY

When the gynecologist becomes more familiar with flexible hysteroscopy, some minor operative procedures can be performed easily without risks.

Removal of intrauterine devices

If the IUD string is lifted into the uterine cavity, it is easy to pull down with a forceps. If the string is broken, we

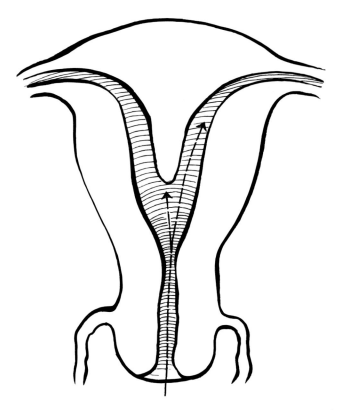

Fig. 8-4. Septum.

choose a grasping forceps. When the IUD is inserted into the endometrium, tools such as the Olympus RG 40 ST or Fuji 3 teeth can be very useful.

It is also possible to remove a lost IUD in early pregnancy. Being able to steer the tip of the endoscope and bypass important structures facilitates observation of the device and its direct removal without compromising the pregnancy.[7]

Polypectomy

Polypectomy is easily performed if the polyp is small or narrow and its pedicle is not too large. The removal can be done using the Olympus lasso, the Fujinon basket, or a Cook alligator forceps. We have not observed any complications or bleeding, and the procedure is painless. The specimen must always be sent to the pathologist for diagnostic confirmation.

Synechiolysis

Synechiolysis is possible only for grade I synechiae, which are thin and filmy. One can use an alligator-type forceps for the adhesiolysis.

Tubal cannulation

Use of a 4.8-mm fiberhysteroscope simplifies hysteroscopy and facilitates fallopian tube cannulation. A 1-mm catheter and its wire guide is used for this purpose. When anatomic variations of the uterine configuration make tubal localization difficult, the flexible hysteroscope is an excellent tool for maneuverability.

DIRECTED OFFICE ENDOMETRIAL CYTOLOGY

We believe that the single, most appropriate application of directed cytology is to detect cancer cells. Only about 70% of routinely obtained endometrial cytologies can be interpreted. The other 30% comprise acellular slides or cells insufficient for diagnosis. We use a 3 French cytobrush (Cook) to collect cells from the desired area, even with a liquid distention medium. The brush spreads the collected cells on a slide, and the fixation is the same as for a pap smear.

Of the 167 directed cytologies we have performed, we have observed four positive results for malignancy confirmed by biopsy and one false negative. Because directed cytology is a quick procedure, we recommend using it in conjunction with a directed biopsy when a suspicious area is detected. Negative results have no predictive value.

DIRECTED ENDOMETRIAL BIOPSIES DURING FIBERHYSTEROSCOPY

Main indications

We believe that gynecologists must perform a biopsy if they are involved in any of the situations listed in the following box:

Main indications for targeted endometrial biopsies during office hysteroscopy

1. Confirmation of a grossly pathologic lesion before a surgical procedure
2. Normal uterine cavity with an abnormal endometrial area
3. Suspicious neoformation with a doubtful visual diagnosis
4. Equivocal ultrasound without hysteroscopic visual correlation
5. Abnormal hysterographic area without an obvious hysteroscopic visual correlation
6. Postmenopausal spotting or bleeding without obvious hysteroscopic pathology
7. Detection of an inflammatory endometrial process with a symptomatic IUD
8. Assessment of hormonal status of the endometrium during an investigation for infertility
9. Evaluation of the endometrial ability to receive the ovum in patients on IVF
10. Classification of the type of endometrial hyperplasia: with or without cytologic atypia
11. Re-evaluation after a medical treatment of endometrial hyperplasia
12. Persistent bleeding after progestin therapy for menometrorrhagia
13. Control of the endometrial hormonal balance in symptomatic patients on hormone replacement therapy
14. Symptomatic patients under tamoxefin citrate therapy, with or without an abnormal vaginal sonogram

---

GENERAL CONSIDERATIONS FOR TARGETED ENDOMETRIAL BIOPSIES

Even with an experienced hysteroscopist, visual diagnosis is hazardous and requires pathologic confirmation to become incontestable. Vaginal sonography is helpful but also has its limitations.

Targeted endometrial biopsy (TEB) is an easy procedure that takes only 3 to 5 minutes to perform. Based on our experience with more than 600 TEBs, it is painless and associated with a very low complication rate. The only difficulty is obtaining enough tissue to allow adequate histologic interpretation. For this purpose, we suggest following a strict protocol developed during our 9 years of practice.

We have to deal with microbiopsies because the working channels on office hysteroscopes are narrow. The quantity of tissue that can be removed ranges from 0.86 to 4.85 mm^3. Several types of nozzles currently available allow us to adapt various forceps to the area to be treated or removed or from which biopsy specimens will be taken. Three leading manufacturers—Olympus, Cook, and Fujinon—have put at our disposal a number of flexible biopsy forceps, which were described in Chapter 4.

For the past 8 years, we have conducted and published three successive studies. The first one (1989, $N = 89$) reported an accuracy of the TEB of 80.2%, with 19.9% rejected because the samples were too small for appropriate histologic evaluation.[9] The accuracy reported in the second study (1990, $N = 69$) was 82.2% accuracy, with a 12.4% rate of rejected biopsies.[10] The third evaluation (1992, $N = 210$) concluded with a diagnosis in more than 92% of samples, with a 2.7% rate of rejected biopsies.[11] We are now working on a fourth evaluation, using a strict protocol listed in the box and in Table 8-1.

From our experience, we can assert the following (next page):

Guidelines for microbiopsies

Protocol

The hysteroscopist should be experienced and skilled.
The hysteroscopist should possess good mastery of the macroscopic appearance of intrauterine pathology.
The hysteroscopist should choose the most appropriate forceps for each case.
The hysteroscopist should obtain tissue for biopsy from a selected area in each pathologic lesion.
The hysteroscopist should perform at least three biopsies.
The hysteroscopist should select a pathologist well trained in gynecology and microbiopsy.
The hysteroscopist should complete a sheet with a good description of the hysteroscopic findings. Include the gross appearance, location of the pathology, and sites of the biopsies.

Table 8-1. Microbiopsy: four different procedures and suggested forceps for each

Type of procedure	Suggested flexible forceps	Example of target
Frontal approach	Standard cup or rat tooth	Endometrium
Oblique approach	Alligator or rat tooth with needle	Myoma
Mobile target	Mouse tooth or rat tooth with needle	Misplaced IUDs or polyp
Biopsy with ablation	Alligator or mouse tooth	Polypectomy

Substantial improvement in sensitivity is closely linked to the number of biopsies performed.

The prudent choice of forceps is mandatory to improving the quality of a biopsy. Selecting the correct forceps involves taking into consideration tissue resistance and lesional topography. The chief obstacle to getting a high-quality biopsy remains the size of the specimen. This difficulty can be markedly reduced through good communication between the hysteroscopist and pathologist. The clinical context is even more important when the sample is small. Because size in the number of tissue fragments is directly related to the accuracy of the histologic diagnosis, at least three biopsy specimens must be taken. This act, according to the patients interviewed, is painless.

Once a sample is taken, it must be set before it is sent to the pathology department. The best fixatives, in descending order, are: Bouin's fluid, Lenker or Larnoy solution, and formaldehyde/10% ethanol. These last two fixatives cause excessive tissue retraction. The fixing procedure leads to tissue dehydration, but this negative effect is offset by the spread on the slide. The area measured should remain close to reality.

As previously stated, because the working channels on office hysteroscopes are narrow (1 to 2.2 mm), physicians must work with microbiopsies. The question then becomes, what is the minimum specimen size required to allow a reliable interpretation of the slide? Pathologists have not yet reached a consensus on the minimal histologic criteria necessary to interpret a tissue sample. This goal can be achieved, however. We have already observed in our studies that the percentage of noninterpretable biopsies decreases proportionately as pathologists acquire more experience in gynecology and in working with the smaller tissue samples.

PRACTICAL ADVICE FOR TISSUE SAMPLING

To benefit fully from the practical advice we offer on tissue sampling, the gynecologist must understand the specific possibilities of the fiberscope and take advantage of its flexibility and bending tip capacity. If used in a proper way, the fiberscope can make obtaining biopsy specimens easier, and tissue sampling can always be performed at the site chosen by the gynecologist.

Determining hormonal status

An endometrial study is best conducted on day 20 to 23 of the menstrual cycle. The samples must be taken essentially from the fundus or near the tubal orifices. The isthmic area is unsuitable because of its partial resistance to hormonal impregnation. A biopsy can be easily performed in the isthmic area; but if a functional polyp is suspected in this area, a biopsy generally is pointless because of the partial resistance to hormonal impregnation.

Polyps

Hysteroscopic analysis of the uterine cavity can reveal polyps, which often are present in menopausal women who have irregular bleeding while on hormone replacement therapy. It is useless to take a tissue sample from the fundus; inflammation, common in that area, can distort the tissue interpretation. A diagnosis is easy to make if a biopsy of the entire polyp is done. On the other hand, a sample of fibrous stroma that is abundant in thick-walled vessels may lead to the diagnosis even if the usual pathologic characteristics are not present.

Endometrial hyperplasia

When it remains localized, endometrial hyperplasia can be easily overshadowed by other benign lesions. The thickness of the endometrium can be appraised by direct contact of the hysteroscope with the uterine wall.

Myomata

Some myomata may appear simply as atrophic endometrium or, inversely, of hyperplasia. Diagnosis rests on a homogeneous organization of the muscular fibers.

Adenocarcinomas

As previously stated, adenocarcinomas can have multiple appearances. Experienced hysteroscopists will suspect certain lesions and confirm their suspicion through directed biopsy sampling. Negative results obtained through usual examinations (i.e., cytology and D&C) cannot absolutely rule out adenocarcinoma.

Because of the small size of the biopsy samples, the best way to recover the fragments is to shake the jaws of the forceps in a cup filled with sterile water. Then the samples can be aspirated with a needle and syringe and immersed in the fixative solution.

RESULTS OF MORE THAN 300 OFFICE HYSTEROSCOPIES

In a French study of office hysteroscopies, the study population comprised 367 patients between the ages of 19 and 82. A group of 64 menopausal patients represented 17.5% of the sample studied. The women in this group were between 40 and 82 years old, with a mean age of 55 years. The mean age of patients of childbearing age was 41 years, while the mean age of the whole sample was 44 years.[3]

The 367 patients were selected on condition that their general gynecologic and obstetric history was clearly established, that previous pelvic ultrasound or hysterographic results were less than 6 months old and a detailed report of the examinations was available, and that all patients had undergone an endometrial biopsy during the flexible hysteroscopy.[3]

Analysis of the patients' medical history revealed the presence of a major gynecologic disorder, excluding parity, in 66.7% of cases. The patients were not selected according to the number and type of previous gynecologic incidents; however, comparing their individual histories with lesions found on examination demonstrated the value of targeted screening by flexible hysteroscopy in office practice.

This type of screening is very useful because of the physical characteristics of the fiberscope: atraumatic, with special appropriateness for the uterine physiologic dimensions; lack of distortion of the cervix by virtue of its adjustable extremity; possession of a very high image definition, combined with an unrestricted ability for exploration of the cavity in the presence of deformations or major intracavitary obstructions; and reproducibility. This reliable and reproducible aspect becomes all the more essential when it is associated with the early acquisition of histologic samples.[9]

INDICATIONS FOR FLEXIBLE HYSTEROSCOPY IN OFFICE PRACTICE

The French experience

Of 367 patients, 49.8% underwent flexible hysteroscopy to evaluate abnormal uterine bleeding (menometrorrhagia, postmenopausal metrorrhagia, spotting with an IUD or while receiving an estrogen-progestogen combination).[3]

In 23% of cases, the patients were monitored for fertility disorders and postmenopausal hormonal treatment.

In 20% of the study population, flexible hysteroscopy supplemented an abnormal suprapubic pelvic ultrasound exploration or hysterography.

In 7% of cases, flexible hysteroscopy was performed as part of a preoperative examination and an evaluation of cancer spread.

In the remaining 3%, flexible hysteroscopy was part of a postoperative follow-up protocol for myomectomy, either transabdominally or by endoscopic laser therapy, for cesarean section follow-up, or to remove a known polyp.

International experience

Office flexible hysteroscopy is useful for monitoring common gynecologic conditions. The procedure can be employed in connection with IUD insertion and use. In particular, patients with a history of intolerance to IUDs may benefit from having an endocavitary inspection through hysteroscopy before another device is inserted. An IUD that will be in place for a long time must be examined for its topography and monitored to ascertain its embedment in the mucosa. Office flexible hysteroscopy is indicated in this situation. In addition, the formation of synechiae secondary to endometrial abrasion may be prevented by a postabortion hysteroscopy performed fairly early in association with the insertion of an IUD.[9,12]

Another application of office flexible hysteroscopy is in examining a pregnant woman who has spontaneously aborted. An examination performed during the 2 weeks following miscarriage eliminates the possibility that placental retention will go clinically unnoticed. A retained placenta can sometimes be the source of bone metaplasia.

Hormone replacement therapy for menopausal women is becoming common. Flexible hysteroscopy in the office can be easily repeated to provide histologic specimens when monitoring patients. It can also help ensure the integrity of the cavity before hormonal therapy is prescibed and it allows the effects of treatment to be monitored.

Oncologic indications

Oncologic evaluation occupies a major place in hysteroscopic prevention. The risk of cancer spread during hysteroscopy has often been mentioned in the medical literature but without a factual basis to confirm this potential. The flexibility of the new hysteroscopes, with their relatively atraumatic technologic design, offers a suitable tool in this context.

The various oncologic indications for flexible hysteroscopy include determining the extent of a neoplasm of the uterine cervix, intrauterine monitoring of pelvic radiotherapy, and systematic screening in high-risk patients. It is also indicated in women with known hyperplasia during the perimenopausal period who wish to receive conservative treatment. Finally, the advent of patients receiving tamoxifen for the treatment of mammary adenocarcinoma has been accompanied by the appearance of local endometrial side effects requiring greater endoscopic vigilance.[9,12]

Flexible hysteroscopy has also been used to screen metaplasia within the transitional zone of the vagina and endocervix that is not visible by speculum and colposcopic examination. Because the instruments used are small, flexible hysteroscopy allows a detailed examination of the cervical canal and external cervical os without causing painful distention.

Obstetric indications

We have found that obstetric indications for office flexible hysteroscopy have become more commonplace and include investigating abnormalities at the origin of a retroplacental hematoma or recurrent placenta previa. In addition, patients who have undergone cervical cerclage during their last pregnancy can benefit from hysteroscopic inspection of the endocervix and for lesions that might increase the risks of prenatal death or secondary sterility. We have used the

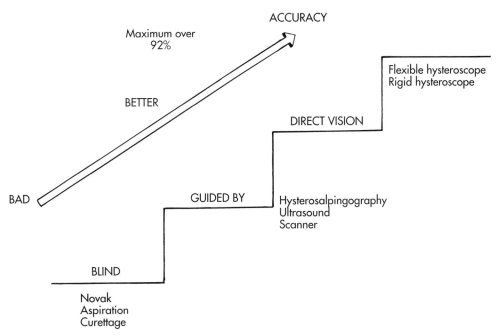

Fig. 8-5. Accuracy of diagnostic modalities to evaluate the endometrial cavity. The specificity of diagnosing endometrial pathology is enhanced by the direct vision provided by office hysteroscopy.

flexible hysteroscope to aid in diagnosing ectopic pregnancy when beta human chorionic gonadotropin levels indicate a nonprogressive pregnancy. The endoscopic examination will often show blackish blood in the tubal ostium.

Indications for minor outpatient surgery

Office surgery remains very restricted in scope and is the province of highly experienced gynecologists who have already performed flexible therapeutic hysteroscopy in the operating theater.

A very good indication for office flexible hysteroscopy is removal of an IUD that is embedded in the endometrium and that cannot be extracted during the initial gynecologic examination. Use of alligator forceps or the Olympus lasso (5 French), or simply coiling the adjustable extremity of the scope may be used to remove the IUDs.

When there are small pedunculated lesions, excisional biopsy is a generally painless and nonhemorrhagic option. It is best performed with a liquid distention medium, which will rinse the cavity, providing better visibility, should slight bleeding occur. Inspection by flexible hysteroscopy is all the more important in oncologic indications in that it enables a supplementary painless histopathologic procedure to occur under direct visual control without increasing operating time.

In the French study by Marty et al,[3] findings from premenopausal patients who had menometrorrhagia were compared with those of Lin,[14,15] who used the same tools through a flexible hysteroscope that Hamou, Wamsteker, and Nargesh[3,16] had used with a rigid endoscope. Biopsies that showed adenocarcinoma ranged between 0.61%

and 5.9% and did not differ statistically from the results in other studies.

Additional indications for office flexible hysteroscopy that are rarely encountered but have been mentioned in the medical literature include examining uterine malformations secondary to diethylstilbesterol exposure in utero, investigating suspected vaginal sarcoma in very young girls, and examining intrauterine lesions indirectly indicative of tubal neoplasia. This last situation was described by an Australian team who discovered a correlation between the presence of periostial yellowish plaques and an asymptomatic endotubal carcinoma without metrorrhagia.

Fig. 8-5 depicts how the specificity of diagnosing endometrial pathology is enhanced by the direct vision provided by office hysteroscopy.

THE ROLE OF FLEXIBLE HYSTEROSCOPY AS A DIAGNOSTIC MODALITY

Mastery of the flexible hysteroscope in conjunction with a supplementary pathologic procedure may suffice in certain situations to obtain an etiologic diagnosis without the need for numerous other examinations. To study the benefits of flexible hysteroscopy compared with other methods of uterine exploration, a comparative analysis of ultrasound diagnoses vs. flexible hysteroscopy and of hysterosalpingographic vs. endoscopic results was conducted.

Comparison of results between echography and flexible hysteroscopy

Of 367 patients examined with flexible hysteroscopy, 167 had a first-line ultrasound scan that disclosed a single

Table 8-2. Hysterographic vs. hysteroscopic findings using rigid and flexible hysteroscopy

Comparative studies

Kessler (1986) *rigid optics*		Marty (1992) *flexible optics*	
Pathologic hysterography			
39% convergent	60% divergent	40% convergent	59% divergent
Total number			
163 cases		52 cases	

Table 8-3. Japanese vs. French findings using flexible hysteroscopy on patients with menometrorrhagia

Comparative studies

	Lin (Japan)	Marty (France)
Normal cavity	189 (42.56%)	79 (44.13%)
Endometrial polyp	51 (11.48%)	51 (28.5%)
Submucous myoma	18 (4.05%)	39 (21.78%)
Endometrial hyperplasia	37 (8.34%)	4 (2.23%)
Synechiae	5 (1.47%)	0
Adenocarcinoma	12 (2.7%)	2 (1.7%)
Number of cases	444	179

lesion. Of these 167 patients, 150 were clearly defined and comprised 38 normal uterine cavities, 79 cases of myoma, 24 cases of endometrial hyperplasia, and 9 cases of fundal polyps. The remaining 17 ultrasound cases were inconclusive.

Diagnostic flexible hysteroscopy performed as a second-line office evaluation confirmed pathology in only 86 of 167 cases, or 51.7%. Of the 17 cases not clearly defined by ultrasound, the following diagnoses were established by flexible hysteroscopy: six normal cavities (of which two had an atrophic endometrium), six submucous myomata, four intracavitary pedunculated polyps, and one endometrial hyperplasia.

Of the 150 cases clearly defined by ultrasound, the diagnoses of single lesions in 86 patients were confirmed by hysteroscopy. Moreover, 62 additional lesions were found that were not detected by ultrasound. These lesions comprised 9 interstitial and submucous myomata, 15 cases of endometrial hyperplasia, 33 polyps, and 5 synechiae.

In 64 cases a multilesional state was underestimated by suprapubic pelvic echography. Of 219 cases explored for cycle disorders, 8.2% false negatives were noted on ultrasound, and 20.5% false positives were noted using the same diagnostic method.

Second-line flexible hysteroscopy supported by pathology corrected the diagnosis in 42.4% of cases. Combined with the false positives, this result increases the discrepancy between these two diagnostic methods to 63%. The sensitivity of suprapubic pelvic ultrasound is on the order of 82%, while the specificity is only 31%. For the past 2 years, we have used only vaginal ultrasound, and both the sensitivity and the specificity have improved.

Comparison of results between hysterography and flexible hysteroscopy

Of 52 hysterographies (HSG) recorded, 21 (40%) yielded results consistent with those obtained by flexible hysteroscopy. Twenty-seven percent of the hysterographies were falsely positive when later examined by hysteroscopy. In 75% of cases in which the specific diagnosis of synechiae was elicited by HSG, the diagnosis was not confirmed by endoscopy. A similar study was performed by Kessler and Lancet[17] with a rigid hysteroscope. The conclusions were similar and proved the superiority of endoscopy (visual inspection) in diagnosing intrauterine lesions (Table 8-2).

In 18 patients who underwent ultrasound, hysterography, and hysteroscopy as part of the exploration for infertility, there was agreement between at least two modalities in 86.5% of cases. There was agreement of all three modalities in only 22% of cases.

INTERNATIONAL EXPERIENCE WITH DIAGNOSTIC FLEXIBLE HYSTEROSCOPY

Diagnostic flexible hysteroscopy is a reliable and reproducible technique offering comparable results in similarly designed independent studies.

The results of our French study were similar to those of the Japanese study by Lin et al,[7,14,15] who examined 444 premenopausal patients with menometrorrhagia using flexible hysteroscopy. Table 8-3 summarizes the data from these studies.

In menopausal patients with spotting, 25 of 52 patients in the French study (48%) and 28 of 67 patients in the Japanese study (41.8%) had a strictly normal hysteroscopic examination and might have otherwise risked undergoing a preventive hysterectomy if not for the precise diagnosis obtained with the office flexible hysteroscope.

One advantage of office flexible hysteroscopy is that it is a reliable examination that provides immediate pathologic findings. An additional advantage provided by the examination is that it is reproducible insofar as it is well tolerated by the patient, which almost guarantees its usefulness in office evaluation and screening.

An American study conducted by Bradley and Widricht[1] under conditions similar to the French study sought to determine patient tolerance to flexible hysteroscopy on the following scale: 1 = easily acceptable discomfort or minimal discomfort; 2 = acceptable discomfort, uncomfortable but easily bearable; 3 = tolerable discomfort, equivalent to menstrual cramps and spasms; 4 = barely touchable, tolerable for a short time only; and 5 = intolerable pain, bad enough to stop the procedure.

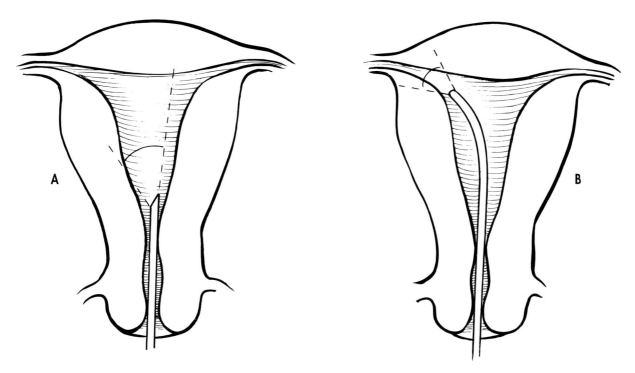

Fig. 8-6. Directed light comparing rigid and flexible hysteroscopy. **A,** The lens of the rigid hysteroscope is fixed at an angle of 30°. **B,** The flexible hysteroscope, with the 0° lens, which can be deflected from 0° to 120°.

Acceptance of the procedure, corresponding to the first three groups, was found in 84% of patients, while 12.4% accepted the conditions of the procedure for a short period (group 4), and 3.6% stopped the procedure because of intolerable pain. The results of this American study were comparable to the French experience.

FLEXIBLE HYSTEROSCOPY VS. RIGID HYSTEROSCOPY

Mechanics

As demonstrated in Fig. 8-6, the principal difference between rigid and flexible hysteroscopy is the ability to deflect the distal extremity of the flexible hysteroscope. This feature allows for a less painful manipulation through the endocervical canal and greater maneuverability within the uterine cavity.

Table 8-4 summarizes the technical differences between flexible and rigid hysteroscopes.

With flexible hysteroscopy there is little or no need to dilate the cervical os. The scope allows frontal observation of a lesion regardless of any cavitary obstruction and the taking of biopsy specimens under direct visual control. Given these technical advantages, we believe the arguments in favor of using a flexible rather than a rigid hysteroscope are irrefutable.

Procedure of rigid hysteroscopy vs. flexible hysteroscopy

In general, performing a hysteroscopic examination with a flexible scope is far less traumatic to the patient than with a rigid scope because of the flexible scope's narrow outer diameter and maneuverable distal extremity.

Unlike the rigid hysteroscope, the diagnostic flexible hysteroscope has a working channel that enables tissue sampling to be performed for biopsy, thus allowing more information to be obtained during a single examination. These factors are summarized in Table 8-5.

DIAGNOSTIC RESULTS WITH FLEXIBLE AND RIGID HYSTEROSCOPES

When flexible hysteroscopy was in its infancy, one of the commonly heard arguments against it was its limited range of vision and poor clarity. Today, however, the optics have been greatly improved, with the reduction of each fiber to 6 to 10 μm, which allows more fibers to be placed within the scope. The result is greater illumination with a smaller diameter. In addition, the moiré filter eliminates the honeycomb appearance, producing an image as clear as that with rigid scopes.

As with any new flexible endoscopic procedure, before being able to correctly determine the topography of abnormal lesions, physicians must first acquire new spatial landmarks by becoming experienced at using the adjustable end coupled with the flexible sheath. At the onset of the examination, the gynecologist must be able to adjust the optics of the endoscope and regulate the luminosity of the cold light and the video camera. No air bubbles or water bubbles should be present between the optics and the head of the video camera.

Once all these steps have been checked, as they need also to be with rigid endoscopes, the argument that optical defi-

Table 8-4. Technical differences between rigid and flexible hysteroscopes

Parameter	Hysteroscopes	
	Rigid	Flexible
External diameter of therapeutic scopes	5.5-7 mm	4.9 mm
External diameter of diagnostic scopes	3.2-5 mm	3.5 mm
Image transfer	Prism system	Fiber optics: transfer of information possible at all angles
Light transfer	Fiber optics	Fiber optics
Distal extremity	Fixed	Adjustable
Intermediate segment	Attached to proximal end	Rotation of 90° on axis (Fujinon only)
Endpiece	Fixed, 12°, 30°, 70°	Flexible, 0°
Angle of field	30°	Therapeutic: 120°
		Diagnostic: 90°
Vision	Oblique, lateral	Frontal

Table 8-5. Clinically relevant differences between rigid and flexible hysteroscopy

Parameter	Hysteroscopes	
	Rigid	Flexible
Cervical dilatation (diagnostic endoscopy)	Commonly necessary	Rarely necessary
Cervical dilatation (therapeutic endoscopy)	Universal	Necessary in 25% of cases
Paracervical anesthesia	Commonly used	Used only with cervical dilatation
Tenaculum	Universal	Rare
Risk of uterine perforation	Possible	Nearly impossible
Reproducibility	Controversial	Documented

Table 8-6. Endocavitary exploration for menometrorrhagia, comparison of findings with rigid and flexible endoscopy*

Comparative studies

	Hamou Rigid	Siegler Rigid	Sciarra Rigid	Barbot Rigid	Wamsteker Rigid	Nargesh Rigid	Marty Flexible
Normal cavity	9 (5%)	15 (42%)	30 (29%)	30 (14%)	85 (41%)	124 (34%)	79 (44%)
Polyp	15 (9%)	10 (28%)	42 (41%)	34 (19%)	39 (20%)	66 (18%)	51 (28%)
Submucous myoma	49 (29%)	6 (17%)	18 (18%)	44 (20%)	16 (8%)	42 (11%)	39 (22%)
Endometrial hyperplasia	39 (24%)	0	4 (4%)	42 (20%)	25 (13%)	85 (23%)	18 (10%)
Atrophy	24 (15%)	0	0	3 (1.5%)	20 (10%)	6 (1.5%)	4 (2%)
Synechiae	0	1 (3%)	2 (2%)	0	3 (1.5%)	21 (6%)	0
Endometrial carcinoma	1 (1%)	0	0	0	12 (6%)	5 (1.3%)	
Uterine malformation	0	1 (3%)	4 (4%)	0		11 (3%)	2 (1%)
Number of cases	164	36	104	213	199	370	179

*The diagnoses of lesions do not diverge when classified into eight homogeneous headings.

nition with a flexible hysteroscope is inferior to that with a rigid hysteroscope is unjustified.

In the recent American study,[1] 71 patients underwent hysterectomy after flexible hysteroscopy. A diagnostic analysis of this method compared with the pathology findings revealed 100% sensitivity and 96% specificity.

A comparative study of hysteroscopic exploration for menometrorrhagia is presented in Table 8-6. In this very common indication, the standard rigid endoscopic interpretation was compared with that of our study, which used flexible endo-

scopes only. The interval between the first and last studies was less than 15 years. There was no statistical difference in the prevalence of intrauterine pathology diagnosed with the rigid and flexible hysteroscopes. The diagnostic precision was as great with flexible endoscopes as with rigid hysteroscopes.[3]

ECONOMIC ADVANTAGES OF FLEXIBLE ENDOSCOPY

Flexible hysteroscopy in office practice is both time and cost effective. Because the procedure is usually performed without general or local anesthesia, no time is required for anesthesiologic consultation or application. In addition, other time-consuming invasive examinations, such as hysterosalpingography, can often be avoided. The time involved in the gynecologic examination, ambulatory endoscopy, and postexploration rest period of 20 to 60 minutes is considerably less than that involved with a 48-hour hospital stay.

The lack of anesthesia makes the patient more independent and eliminates the need for a postexamination attendant, allowing physicians to retain a limited office staff.

In the United States, the average patient charge for ambulatory flexible hysteroscopy is estimated to be $475 vs. $3495 for in-hospital diagnostic hysteroscopy.[1]

CONCLUSION

Flexible hysteroscopy is a safe, simple, and cost-effective procedure that can be used for screening target populations. It permits early, accurate diagnosis of intrauterine pathology, which can then be confirmed with histologic accuracy. This ability in itself obviates the need for expensive and less accurate testing such as blind D&Cs. The short learning curve associated with performing office flexible hysteroscopy can help this procedure become an integral part of the armamentarium of all gynecologists and primary health care providers.

REFERENCES

1. Bradley LD, Widricht T: State of the art of flexible hysteroscopy for office gynecologic evaluation, *Journal of the American Association of Gynecologic Laparoscopists* 2(3):263-267, 1995.
2. Parent B et al: Hysteroscopie panorathique. Maloine SA, Ed: 1985.
3. Mussuto P: The challenges of flexibility in hysteroscopy: its diagnostic and therapeutic contributions in obstetrics and gynecology, Future Prospects, Thesis PA 060032, 1993. Faculté de Médecine, Broussais Hotel-Dieu, France, 1993.
4. Peterson WF, Novak E: Endometrial polyps, *Obstet Gynecol* 8:4049, 1956.
5. DeBrux J: Hystopathologie gynecologique, Masson, W, Ed: Paris, 1982.
6. Sugimoto O, Ushiroyama T, Fukuda Y: In Siegler AM, Lendimann HJ, Eds: *Hysteroscopy: principles and practice,* ed 3, Philadelphia, 1984, Lippincott.
7. Lin BL et al: Outcome of removal of intrauterine devices with flexible hysteroscopy in early pregnancy, *J Gynecol Surg* 9:995, 1993.
8. Marty R, Valle RF: Hysteroscopic procedures with flexible fiberscopes: eight years experience, *Journal of the American Association of Gynecologic Laparoscopists* 3(1):113-118, 1995.
9. Marty R et al: The reliability of endometrial biopsy performed during hysteroscopy, *Int J Gynecol Obstet* 31:151-155, 1990.
10. Marty R et al: Endometrial biopsy during office hysteroscopy with a three French flexible biopsy forceps: evaluation of over 69 cases. AAGL International Congress, *Book of abstracts: new instrumentation,* 1990, p 157.
11. Marty R, Amouroux J, DeBrux J: The targeted endometrial biopsy during flexible hysteroscopy: technic and results, International Congress of Gynecologic Endoscopy, Seoul, Korea, Book of Abstracts, L25:61, 1992.
12. Karacz B: Office hysteroscopy. In Siegler AM, Lendimann HJ, Eds: *Hysteroscopy: principles and practice,* ed 3, Philadelphia, 1984, Lippincott.
13. Miyazawa K: Selective use of hysteroscopy in gynecologic oncology. In Siegler AM, Lendimann HJ, Eds: *Hysteroscopy: principles and practice,* ed 3, Philadelphia, 1984, Lippincott.
14. Lin BL, Imata Y, Jomamatsu M: The development of a new flexible hysteroscope and its clinical application, *Acta Obstet Gynecol* LPN, 36:659, 1985.
15. Lin BL et al: The Fujinon diagnostic fiber optic hysteroscope experience with 1503 patients, *J Reprod Med* 35(7):685-689, 1990.
16. Nargesh Q, Motashaw ND, Svati D: Diagnostic and therapeutic hysteroscopy in the management of abnormal uterine bleeding, *J Reprod Med* 36(6):616-620, 1990.
17. Kessler I, Lancet M: Hysterography and hysteroscopy: a comparison, *Fertil Steril* 464:709-710, 1986.

Chapter 9

CASE PRESENTATIONS AND COMMON PATHOLOGY DIAGNOSED WITH OFFICE HYSTEROSCOPY

John Bertrand

CASE 1. NORMAL UTERINE CAVITY

P.W. is 57-year-old G_2P_{2002} postmenopausal female with no history of abnormal vaginal bleeding. She had a vaginal probe ultrasound performed as a screening test before being placed on hormone replacement therapy. Her endometrium was felt to be thickened at 10 mm, and she was referred for hysteroscopic evaluation. The procedure was performed using a 3.6-mm flexible hysteroscope and normal saline for uterine distention.

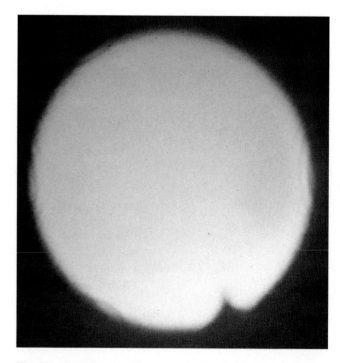

A

Fig. 9-1. A, Before instilling normal saline for distention, the hysteroscopist gently places the instrument within the cervical canal in the straight position until resistance is noted.

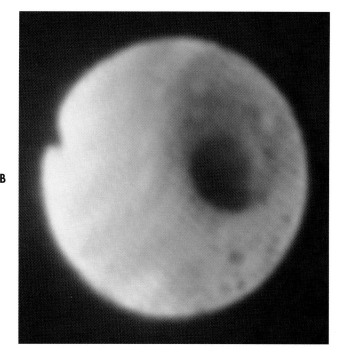

Fig. 9-1. B, The saline is instilled with a 60-ml syringe, and the hysteroscope is withdrawn slightly until the internal cervical ostium is visualized. At this point the hysteroscope should be advanced into the endometrial cavity using a no-touch technique, keeping the opening to the cavity in the center of the picture.

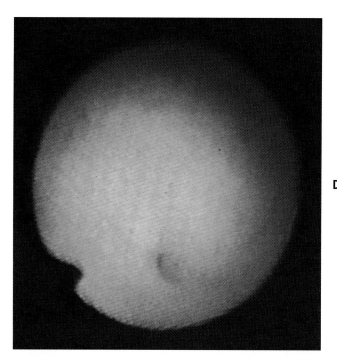

Fig. 9-1. D, Visualization of the left tubal ostium.

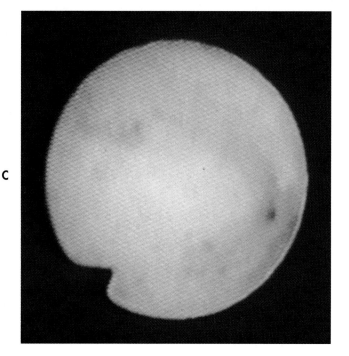

Fig. 9-1. C, Visualization of the right tubal ostium.

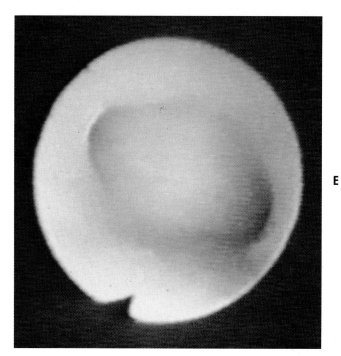

Fig. 9-1. E, Panoramic view of the endometrial cavity from the internal cervical ostium.

CASE 2. INTRAUTERINE SYNECHIAE

R.S. is a 34-year-old G_1P_{0010} female with a 2-year history of secondary infertility. Her history is significant for an elective abortion at age 18. There was no history of pelvic inflammatory disease, endometritis, or use of an intrauterine contraceptive device. The infertility workup included a biphasic basal body temperature chart, normal semen analysis, in-phase endometrial biopsy, normal postcoital test, and hysterosalpingogram demonstrating bilateral proximal tubal occlusion. The patient elected to proceed directly to in vitro fertilization and as part of the routine workup, an office hysteroscopic examination was performed.

The following six slides were taken using the Olympus HYF-P (3.6-mm) flexible hysteroscope and CO_2 distention.

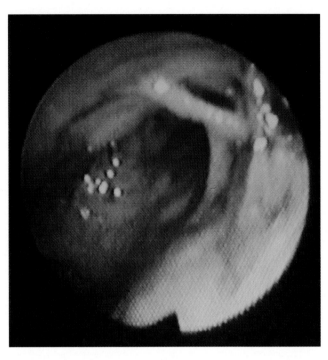

Fig. 9-2. B, Panoramic view of the uterine cavity from the internal cervical ostium looking toward the uterine fundus. This is the best position to visualize macroscopic pathology, such as submucous fibroids, endometrial polyps, or synechiae as demonstrated here.

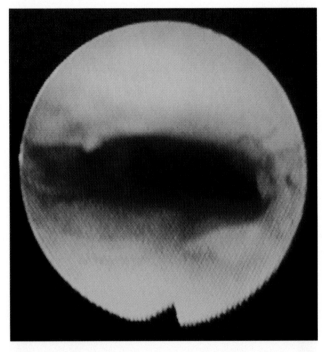

Fig. 9-2. A, View of the internal cervical ostium from the cervical canal. The flexible hysteroscope is advanced through the cervical canal, keeping this landmark in the middle of the optical field. The progression should be done using a no-touch technique, meaning the hysteroscope should be advanced while making an effort not to allow the distal tip to touch the cervical sidewalls.

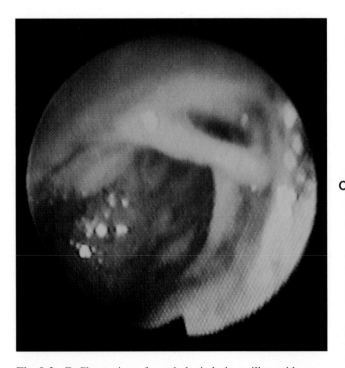

Fig. 9-2. C, Closer view of a pathologic lesion will provide magnification of the lesion. This can be done with most flexible hysteroscopes without having to refocus the image. A closeup view of this lesion demonstrates the avascular appearance typical of intrauterine synechiae.

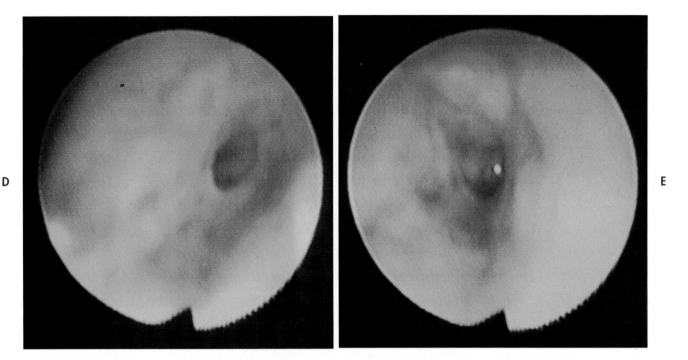

Figs. 9-2. D and **E,** To ensure complete visualization of the entire uterine cavity, both tubal ostia should be seen as demonstrated in these two photographs. If one or the other ostium is not visualized, it should be recorded in the patient's chart that the examination was incomplete and that additional intrauterine pathology cannot be ruled out.

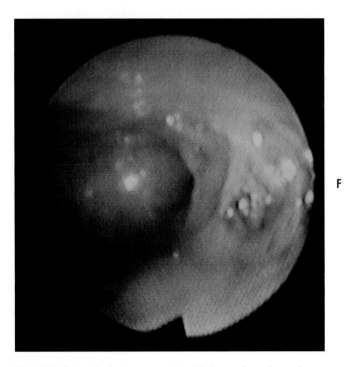

Fig. 9-2. F, As the hysteroscope is withdrawn from the endometrial cavity, the hysteroscopist should complete a last panoramic view of the cavity. The same should be done of the cervical canal as the hysteroscope is slowly withdrawn into the vagina.

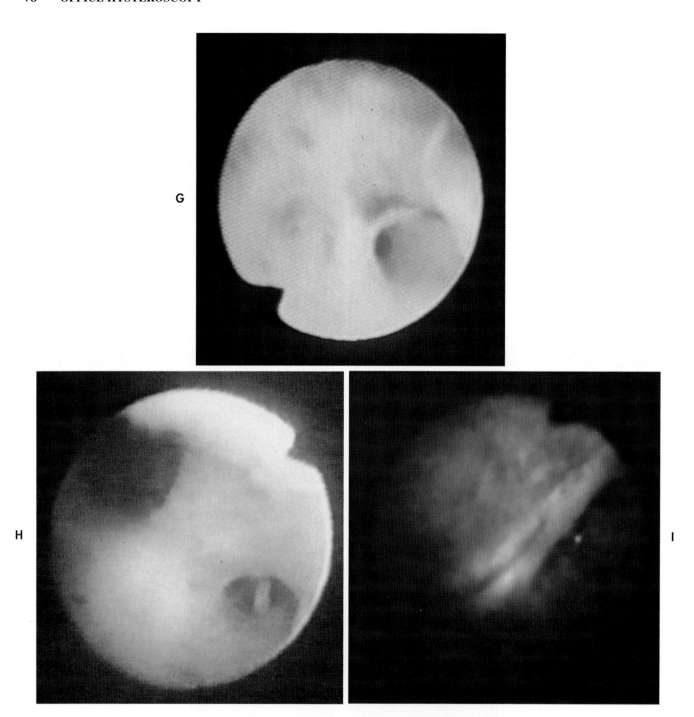

Fig. 9-2. G, Examples of synechiae within the cervix **(G)** and miduterine segment **(H),** and on the fundal wall **(I),** as viewed with a 3.6-mm flexible hysteroscope using normal saline for uterine distention.

CASE 3. ATYPICAL ENDOMETRIAL HYPERPLASIA

R.P. is a 51-year-old G_2P_{2002} postmenopausal female who experienced irregular vaginal bleeding for 3 weeks. The patient had been on estrogen replacement therapy without progestins for 18 months.

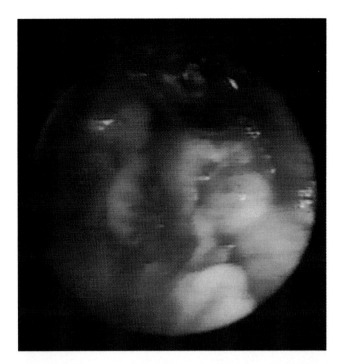

Fig. 9-3. An office hysteroscopic examination was performed using a flexible 3.6-mm hysteroscope and CO_2 for uterine distention. A biopsy of the hemorrhagic area in the middle of the figure showed atypical endometrial hyperplasia.

CASE 4. ENDOMETRIAL POLYPS

P.L. is a 39-year-old G_2P_{2002} female with metrorrhagia. Her regular cycles were every 28 to 30 days; however, she experienced midcycle spotting as well. A midcycle blind endometrial biopsy was performed and showed secretory endometrium consistent with cycle day 17 to 18. She was given a trial of oral contraceptives and progestin therapy, neither of which controlled her irregular bleeding.

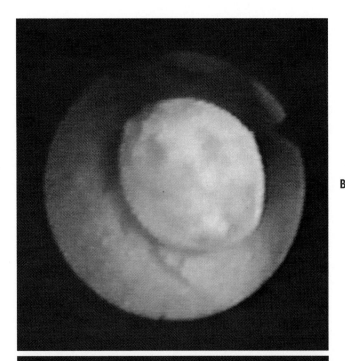

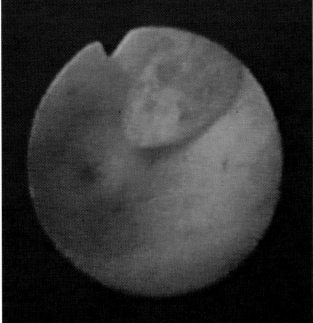

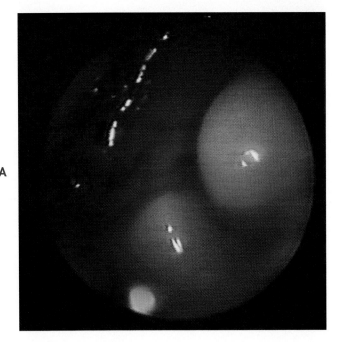

Fig. 9-4. A, An office hysteroscopic examination was performed with a 4.9-mm flexible hysteroscope using CO_2 for uterine distention. Two polyps were discovered on the uterine sidewalls, and they were subsequently removed.

Figs. 9-4 B and **C.** Additional examples of endometrial polyps viewed through a 3.6-mm flexible hysteroscope using normal saline for uterine distention. **B,** Polyp originating on the posterior uterine wall. **C,** Polyp near the right tubal ostium.

CASE 5. ADENOMYOSIS

A.C. is a 35-year-old G_0 female with a 2-year history of infertility, as well as worsening hypermenorrhea and dysmenorrhea. Her infertility workup included biphasic basal body temperature charts, in-phase endometrial biopsy, a normal semen analysis, postcoital test, and histosalpingogram. Laparoscopy revealed stage II endometriosis.

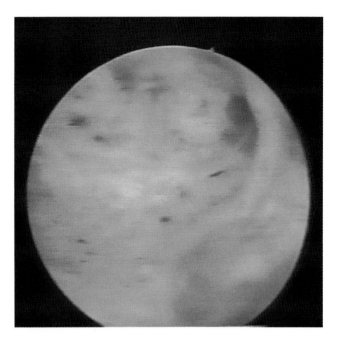

Fig. 9-5. An office hysteroscopic examination was performed using a 4.9-mm flexible hysteroscope. There was diffuse pitting of the endometrium into the myometrium, suggesting the presence of adenomyosis. A pelvic MRI subsequently obtained demonstrated diffuse thickening of the junctional zone, a finding consistent with adenomyosis.

CASE 6. SEPTATE UTERUS

C.W. is a 27-year-old G_2P_{0020} female who had a 1-year history of secondary infertility, as well as a history of two first-trimester spontaneous miscarriages. In addition, there was a questionable history of in-utero exposure to diethylstilbestrol.

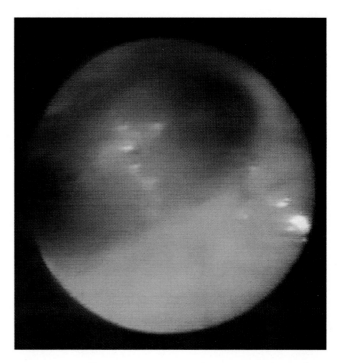

Fig. 9-6. An office hysteroscopic examination was performed using a 3.6-mm flexible hysteroscope and CO_2 for uterine distention. A large midline defect was noted, which was consistent with either a uterine septum or a bicornuate uterus. Laparoscopy subsequently confirmed a uterine septum, and this was repaired with an operative hysteroscope.

CASE 7. ENDOCERVICAL POLYP

D.B. is a 32-year-old G_1P_1 female with a 6-month history of postcoital bleeding. All of her pap smears have been normal, and on physical examination of the cervix there were no gross lesions or ectropion.

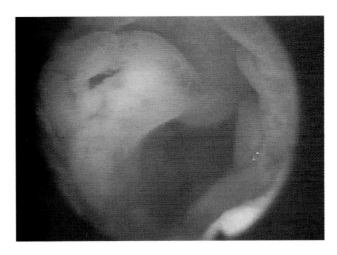

Fig. 9-7. An office hysteroscopic examination was performed using a 4.9-mm flexible hysteroscope and normal saline for uterine distention. An endocervical polyp was diagnosed and removed in the office with flexible alligator forceps under direct visualization.

CASE 8. ENDOMETRIAL ADENOCARCINOMA

L.T. is a 41-year-old G_0 female referred for endometrial ablation. She had a 6-month history of menorrhagia unresponsive to oral contraceptives and nonsteroidal antiinflammatory agents. An endometrial biopsy revealed proliferative endometrium.

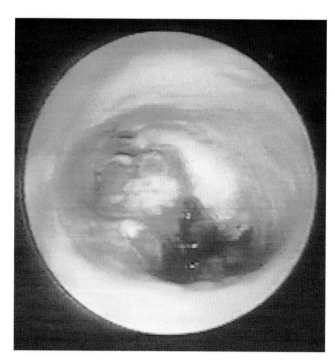

Fig. 9-8. An office hysteroscopic examination was performed using a 3.6-mm flexible hysteroscope and CO_2 for uterine distention. A directed biopsy of the focal lesion seen in the lower uterine segment revealed it to be a grade I-II endometrial adenocarcinoma.

CASE 9. ADENOMYOSIS

W.S. is a 51-year-old G_6P_{6006} postmenopausal female on cyclic hormone replacement therapy who had heavy uterine bleeding and anemia. When the hormone replacement therapy was discontinued, the bleeding ceased; however, the patient suffered from severe vasomotor symptoms. An endometrial biopsy revealed slightly proliferative endometrium. A sonohysterographic examination was normal.

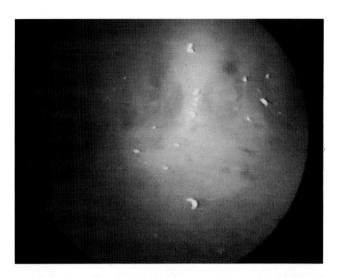

Fig. 9-9. An office hysteroscopic examination was performed using a 3.6-mm flexible hysteroscope and CO_2 for uterine distention. Numerous pits noted in the endometrium were found to be extending into the myometrium, suggesting extensive adenomyosis. This diagnosis was confirmed following a hysterectomy.

CASE 10. SUBMUCOUS FIBROID

A.C. is a 47-year-old G_2P_{2002} female with a 9-month history of menometrorrhagia. Her evaluation included a normal vaginal probe ultrasound and endometrial biopsy. Her basal body temperature charts demonstrated irregular ovulation so she was given a trial of oral contraceptives, which cleared her metrorrhagia, but she continued to suffer from heavy periods.

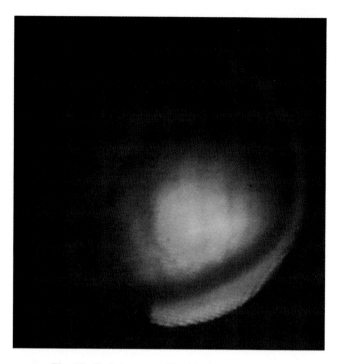

Fig. 10. B, Submucous fibroid with a broad base.

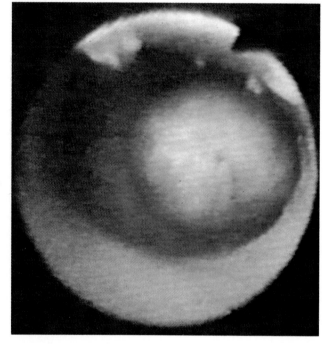

Fig. 9-10. A, An office hysteroscopic examination was performed using a 3.6-mm flexible hysteroscope and normal saline for distention. A 2.5-cm pedunculated submucous fibroid was seen with its stalk near the left cornua.

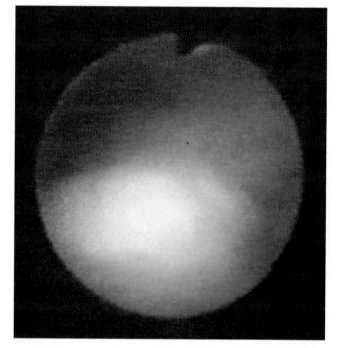

Fig. 10. C, Fibroid that is approximately 30% submucous and 70% intramural. This information is helpful during preoperative planning.

CASE 11. UTERINE SEPTUM

J.I. is a 27-year-old G_3P_{0030} female with a 2-year history of secondary infertility. She has been able to conceive spontaneously without difficulty; however, each pregnancy has ended in a first-trimester miscarriage. Her workup included normal levels of thyroid-stimulating hormone and prolactin, negative cervical cultures, in-phase endometrial biopsy, normal maternal and paternal karyotypes, and a negative antiphospholipid antibody profile.

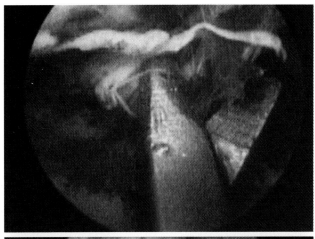

C

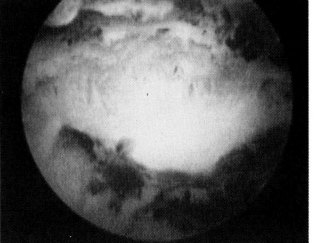

D

Figs. 9-11 C and **D.** Following a pelvic MRI, which demonstrated that the uterine defect was a septum and not a bicornuate uterus, hysteroscopic resection of the uterine septum was performed with a continuous-flow 24 French operating hysteroscope and semi-rigid scissors. Normal saline was used for uterine distention.

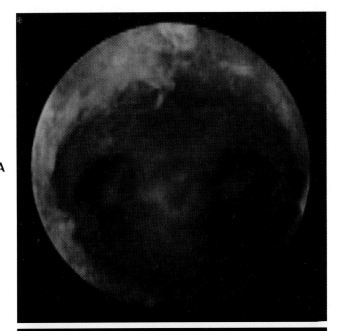

A

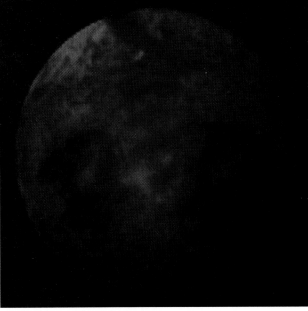

B

Figs. 9-11 A and **B.** An office hysteroscopic examination was performed using a 4.9-mm flexible hysteroscope and normal saline for distention. **A,** Panoramic view of the endometrial cavity. **B,** Closeup of the uterine septum.

CASE 12. SUBMUCOUS FIBROID

A.G. is a 42-year-old G_2P_{2002} female with a 1-year history of heavy uterine bleeding. Her evaluation included a biphasic basal body temperature chart and endometrial biopsy that showed secretory endometrium. Clotting studies and platelet function studies were also performed because of a history of aspirin abuse, but results were normal.

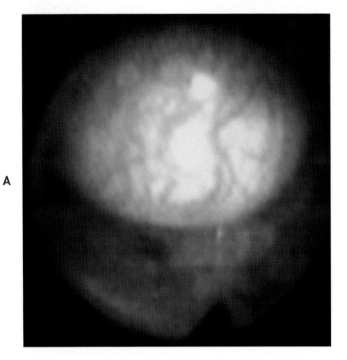

Fig. 9-12. A, Flexible hysteroscopy was performed using a 3.6-mm fiberscope and normal saline for uterine distention. A 2-cm submucous fibroid on a stalk was found in the right uterine cornu.

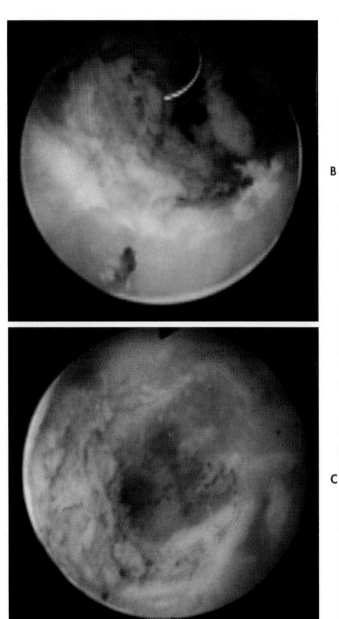

Fig. 9-12 B and **C.** Hysteroscopic resection of a uterine fibroid using a 27 French resectoscope, wire loop, and 1.5% glycine for uterine distention. The procedure was performed in the operating room under general anesthesia.

CASE 13. SUBMUCOUS FIBROID

N.I. is a 44-year-old G_3P_{3003} female with severe menorrhagia and anemia. Her medical history was significant for spontaneous deep-vein thrombosis requiring long-term anticoagulation therapy. Her religious beliefs prevented her from accepting blood transfusions. Her evaluation included an endometrial biopsy, which revealed secretory endometrium.

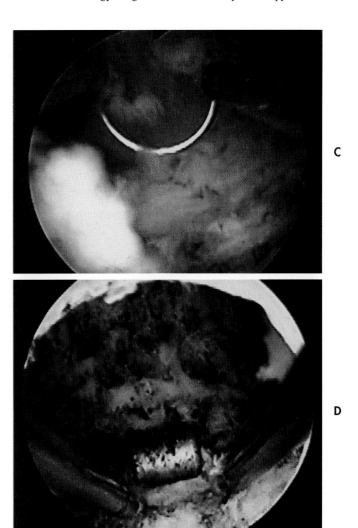

Figs. 9-13 C and **D.** In the operating room and under general anesthesia, the submucous fibroids were resected (**C**) using a wire loop through a 27 French continuous-flow resectoscope. **D,** After the fibroid resection was completed, the remainder of the endometrial cavity was ablated with a "roller bar."

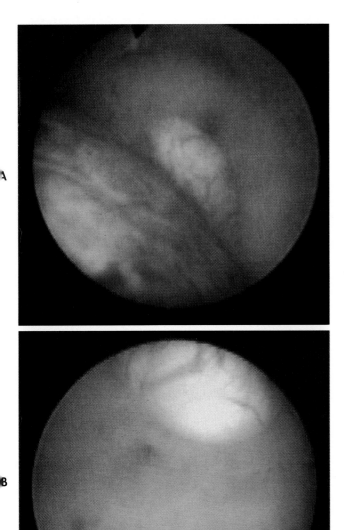

Figs. 9-13 A and **B.** An office hysteroscopic examination was performed using a 3.6-mm flexible hysteroscope and normal saline for uterine distention. **A,** View behind a large submucous fibroid, which demonstrates a smaller fibroid and the left tubal ostium. **B,** View of the right tubal ostium and another small submucous fibroid. These photographs illustrate the importance of viewing both tubal ostia for a complete hysteroscopic evaluation.

CASE 14. PROXIMAL TUBAL RECANALIZATION

V.P. is a 28-year-old G_2P_{0020} female with a 2-year history of secondary infertility. Her medical history is significant for a severe episode of pelvic inflammatory disease following her last D&C. Treatment required hospitalization and intravenous antibiotics. Since this episode, her menstrual flow has been reduced. A hysterosalpingogram revealed suspected adhesions in the right cornual area, as well as bilateral proximal tubal obstruction.

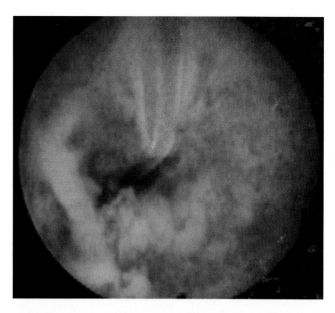

B

Fig. 9-14. B, A 3 French Novy catheter placed through the 2.2-mm working channel of a 4.9-mm flexible hysteroscope has been advanced through the interstitial portion of the right fallopian tube to clear the proximal tubal obstruction.

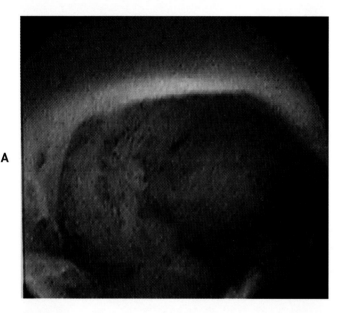

A

Fig. 9-14. A, An office hysteroscopic examination was performed with a 4.9-mm flexible hysteroscope and normal saline for uterine distention. This figure demonstrates occlusion of the right cornual region of the endometrial cavity.

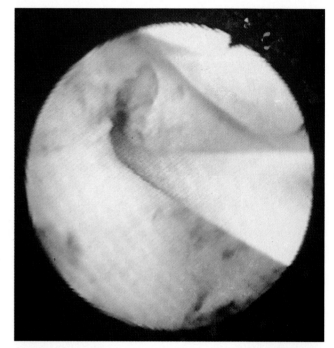

C

Fig. 9-14. C, Another example of proximal tubal recanalization. In this case a 0.032-inch Teflon-coated guidewire has been extended through the 2.2-mm working channel of a 4.9-mm flexible hysteroscope.

CASE 15. ENDOMETRIAL ADENOCARCINOMA

M.M. is a 44-year-old G_0 female with a 2-year history of menometrorrhagia. She has a history of poorly controlled diabetes mellitus due to poor patient compliance. An endometrial biopsy revealed grade I-II endometrial adenocarcinoma.

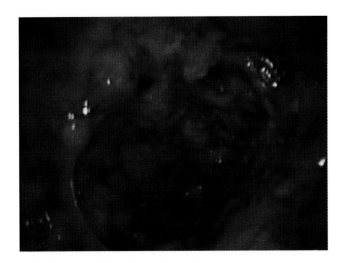

Fig. 9-15. An office hysteroscopic examination performed using a 4.9-mm flexible hysteroscope and CO_2 for uterine distention reveals an endometrial carcinoma that has involved the entire endometrial cavity.

CASE 16. ENDOMETRIAL POLYP

N.S. is a 35-year-old G_0 female with a 2-year history of primary infertility. A hysterosalpingogram was performed and suggested a filling defect in the right cornu. The left tube was patent, but the right tube demonstrated proximal obstruction.

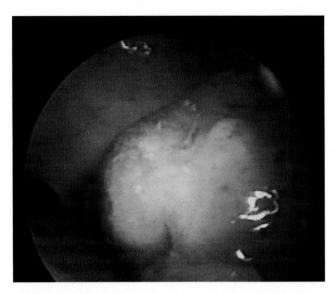

Fig. 9-16. An office hysteroscopic examination performed using a 4.9-mm flexible hysteroscope and CO_2 for uterine distention shows a large endometrial polyp occluding the right tubal ostium. The left tubal ostium is clearly visualized.

CASE 17. PEDUNCULATED SUBMUCOUS FIBROID

V.R. is a 33-year-old G_0 female with a 1-year history of primary infertility, as well as menorrhagia. Her evaluation included a biphasic basal body temperature chart and an in-phase endometrial biopsy.

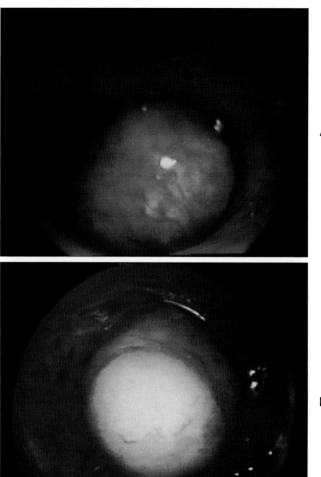

A

B

Figs. 9-17 A and **B.** An office hysteroscopic examination was performed using a 4.9-mm flexible hysteroscope and CO_2 for uterine distention. **A,** Frontal view of a pedunculated fibroid. **B,** Side view of the fibroid.

CASE 18. SECRETORY ENDOMETRIUM

A.W. is a 36-year-old G_0 female who was visiting from out of the country and presented with one episode of unusual heavy vaginal bleeding. Her cycles were irregular. An office hysteroscopic examination was performed on cycle day 36. Her serum β-HCG was negative.

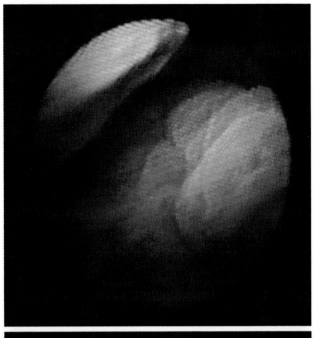

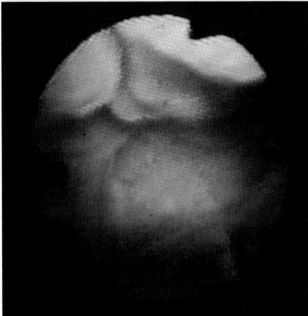

Figs. 9-18 A and **B.** An office hysteroscopic examination was performed using a 3.6-mm flexible hysteroscope and normal saline for distention. The examination was inadequate because of the fluffy secretory endometrium present.

CASE 19. IUD

X.Z. is a 32-year-old G_1P_{1001} female who was visiting from China and had a 6-month history of menometrorrhagia. Because she was in town for only a short time, an office hysteroscopic examination was performed on the day of her first visit.

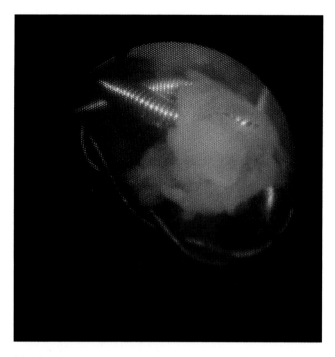

Fig. 9-19. An office hysteroscopic examination was performed using a 4.9-mm flexible hysteroscope and normal saline for distention. A circular IUD was found that had no string and was not known by the patient to be present. Because of the side effects, the patient wanted the IUD taken out. The removal was performed in the office with alligator grasping forceps placed through the working channel of the flexible hysteroscope.

CASE 20. EMBEDDED IUD

C.C. is a 57-year-old G_2P_2 postmenopausal female who requested that her Copper 7 IUD be removed. It had been in place for 16 years and had caused no abnormal symptoms. The string was present within the cervical canal; however, the IUD did not advance even after a vigorous pull. An office hysteroscopic examination was performed to help explain the difficulty in removing the IUD.

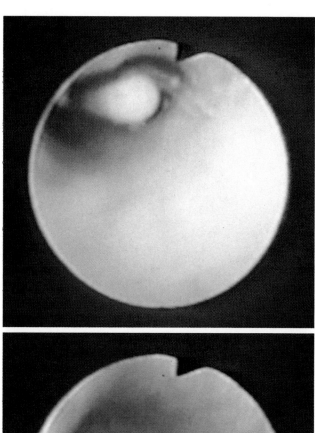

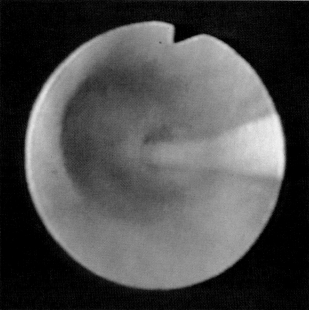

Figs. 9-20 A and **B.** An office hysteroscopic examination was performed using a 3.6-mm flexible hysteroscope and normal saline for uterine distention. **A,** Proximal portion of the IUD within the cervix. **B,** Distal portion exiting the right tubal ostium. The IUD was subsequently removed under laparoscopic guidance to ensure no uterine tears would go unnoticed.

Chapter 10

TECHNIQUES FOR OPERATIVE OFFICE HYSTEROSCOPY

Richard J. Gimpelson

Although diagnostic hysteroscopy has been accepted as an office procedure,[1] operative hysteroscopy still is performed mainly in the hospital or outpatient surgery center. However, many operative hysteroscopies can be performed in an office setting, resulting in a savings of time for the gynecologist and reduction of cost for the patient.[2,3] For safe and successful operative office hysteroscopy, one must know which procedures can be done and how to do them. Success and safety also depend on using the proper equipment and careful patient selection, but operator experience is the most important consideration.

Operative office hysteroscopy enables the physician to diagnose and treat abnormal uterine bleeding secondary to leiomyomas and polyps, identify and remove intrauterine foreign bodies such as IUDs, and in certain circumstances treat infertility and pregnancy wastage.

Between Jan. 1, 1983, and Oct. 1, 1995, the author performed 1872 hysteroscopic procedures. Of these, 832 were performed in the operating room, 938 in the office and 102 in a "hysteroscopy center," a hospital-based facility set up like an office and used primarily when insurance does not cover the cost of office supplies. Approximately 26% of the 1040 office hysteroscopies were operative (Table 10-1).

INDICATIONS

Submucous leiomyomas and polyps can cause abnormal uterine bleeding, infertility, and pregnancy wastage. Many of these lesions can be easily resected in an office setting. Removal of an intrauterine device in which the string is gone or retracted is almost always accomplished in the office with very little need to use an operating room. Intrauterine adhesions can be lysed under certain circumstances in the office

as can tubal canalization to confirm patency or overcome blockage.

Even if no obvious lesion is seen under hysteroscopic examination, one can take tissue for biopsy from raised areas or areas of different color and obtain a diagnosis often missed on blind dilatation and curettage.[4]

CONTRAINDICATIONS

Cervical cancer is the only absolute contraindication to operative office hysteroscopy because hysteroscopic findings add no information for aiding in treatment.[5] Another contraindication is acute pelvic infection, unless it is related to an intrauterine device. Desired pregnancy with an IUD is a third exception. In this case, hysteroscopy should be limited to removal of the device before initating antibiotic therapy.[6] Relative contraindications are extensive adhesions, uterine septa, and leiomyomas more than 2 cm in diameter and less than 50% in the uterine cavity. The medical or mental status of a patient may also be a contraindication to operative office hysteroscopy. Patients with severe diabetes, asthma, and bleeding disorders can have a rapid onset of adverse reactions and may best be treated in the operating room, where problems can be handled by support personnel.

Cervical stenosis and active bleeding have been cited as relative contraindications to hysteroscopic surgery.[7] However, neither of these factors has caused problems in my practice. The uterine cavity can be easily cleared of blood and clots by using a 5-, 6-, or 7-mm suction curette, thus allowing an adequate hysteroscopic procedure to be performed.[8] Cervical stenosis is often significant only at the external os. If one gently dilates the cervical os, a 5-mm diagnostic sheath and telescope often can be easily advanced into the uterine cavity or at least guide dilatation in the proper direction.

INSTRUMENTATION

Although diagnostic hysteroscopy can be done with minimal instrumentation, operative office hysteroscopy requires a large number of instruments (see adjacent box) to enhance successful surgery even though only a small number are used in most procedures.[3,9] The initial examination usually is performed with a rigid 4-mm telescope in a 5-mm sheath. The 2.7-mm telescope with a 3.5-mm sheath and the 3.6-mm flexible hysteroscope are also good for diagnostic hysteroscopy but not for operative hysteroscopy. A 5.5-mm continuous-flow sheath is available for office hysteroscopy with fluids but is limited mainly to diagnostic procedures and very small directed biopsies.

Table 10-1. Office hysteroscopy procedures

Procedure	Number in office	Number in hysteroscopy center
Diagnostic	705	66
Polypectomy (endometrial)	90	14
Myomectomy	70	9
Polypectomy (endocervical)	4	3
Lysis of adhesions	32	3
IUD removal	8	
Follow-up septum (division)	9	
Transcervical sterilization (silicone plugs)	19	
Endometrial ablation (initial)		6
Endometrial ablation (repeat)	1	
Cervical stenosis		1
Total	938	102

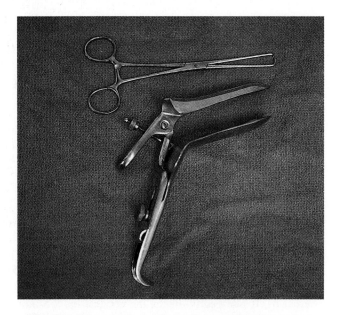

Fig. 10-1. Open-sided speculum and conventional tenaculum.

Light sources can range from relatively inexpensive 150 W tungsten filament projection bulbs to 300 W xenon lights if 35-mm photo documentation is desired. The video cameras and telescopes available today are all sensitive enough to allow a good view even with the 150 W light source.

A CO_2 insufflator is needed if the operative office hysteroscopy is performed with CO_2 as the distention medium. An open-sided speculum and a conventional tenaculum with two teeth are used in most procedures (Fig. 10-1). A four-toothed tenaculum (Fig. 10-2) has been developed to minimize the reflux of distention media in those overdilated or patulous cervices when CO_2 or liquid distention media are used.[10]

Approximate costs of office hysteroscopy setup

4-mm telescope	$3,200.00
5-mm sheath (diagnostic)	475.00
7-mm sheath (operative)	675.00
Flexible scissors	475.00
Flexible forceps	425.00
Flexible grasper	300.00
Semirigid scissors	475.00
Semirigid forceps	475.00
Semirigid grasper	475.00
Rigid scissors	650.00
Rigid forceps	750.00
Rigid grasper	650.00
Light cable	475.00
Light source	
Least expensive	950.00
Xenon (most expensive)	6,000.00
Video camera	5,000.00
Monitor	
Least expensive	200.00
Most expensive	1,000.00
Insufflator	1,860.00
Conventional tenaculum	15.00
Cervical-sealing tenaculum	375.00
Open-sided speculum	37.00
Examination table (electric)	6,000.00
Myoma extractor	250.00
Ring forceps	15.00
Pituitary rongeur	(obtain from neurosurgery)
Emergency kit	775.00
Foley catheter (30-cc balloon)	2.00
Dilators (Pratt)	180.00
Hyskon pump	
Least expensive (60-ml syringe)	1.00
Most expensive	1,600.00
Pulse oximeter	2,500.00
Laser jet printer (for pulse oximeter)	500.00
Suction pump	450.00*
Suction curettes	
Tis-U-Traps (each)	12.00*

*Check with supplier; pump may be free with purchase of 200 or more curettes.

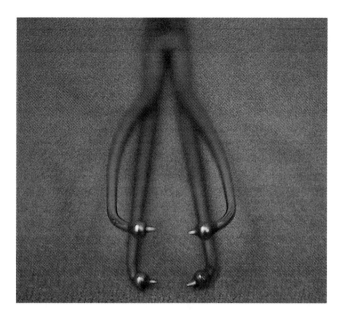

Fig. 10-2. Four-toothed tenaculum. Instrument patent No. 5,059,198 held by Richard J. Gimpelson, M.D., and licensed to Wolf Medical Instruments Corp, Vernon Hills, Ill.

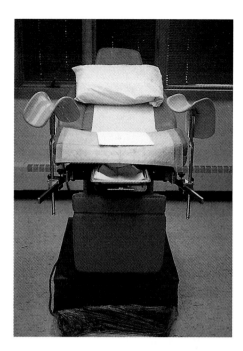

Fig. 10-4. Table with behind-the-knee stirrups.

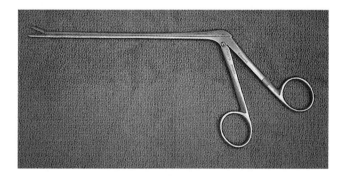

Fig. 10-3. Pituitary rongeur.

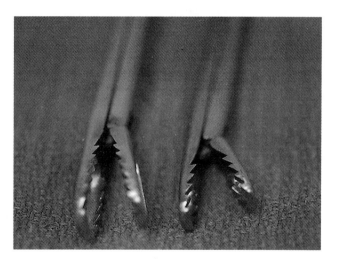

Fig. 10-5. Myoma-grasping forceps.

Obviously an operating hysteroscopy sheath is needed to do operative hysteroscopy. These sheaths are 7 or 8 mm in diameter and use the standard 4-mm telescope. Various 7 French (2-mm) instruments can be inserted through the operating channels of the operating sheath. The 7 French instruments are either flexible or semirigid and are used as biopsy forceps, scissors, or graspers. Rigid instruments are also available that attach to the hysteroscopy sheath by their own bridge, but they are rarely used because the operator must insert the hysteroscope and work with the tips of the instrument always sticking out in front of the telescope. One of the most functional instruments used is a pituitary rongeur (Fig. 10-3), which is inserted into the uterine cavity alongside the diagnostic sheath to resect leiomyomas and polyps or retrieve a lost IUD under direct visualization.

Operative office hysteroscopy is most easily performed with the patient on an electric procedure table with tilting capability. It is best if the table can be elevated to 46 to 48 inches; however, use of a video camera allows the table

height to be lower. The patient's legs are kept comfortable with behind-the-knee stirrups (Fig. 10-4). A ring forceps and myoma-grasping forceps (Fig. 10-5) are employed to remove large lesions, although they often are used blindly because they are difficult to use with a telescope.

The operator must be prepared for emergencies and should keep resuscitation equipment and medication on hand. A Foley catheter with a 30-cc balloon may be used if uncontrolled heavy bleeding occurs. The catheter is inserted in the uterine cavity, and the balloon is inflated to act as both tamponade and drain. This gives the physician time to observe the patient and decide if she is able to go home or needs to be transferred to a hospital.

Because local anesthesia and sedation are often needed for operative hysteroscopy, a pulse oximeter is used to monitor the patient's pulse and oxygen saturation. This allows one to quickly note the bradycardia associated with vasovagal reaction. The pulse oximeter can minimize the chance of respiratory arrest—a most serious complication—by warning of a drop in oxygen saturation.

DISTENTION MEDIA

CO_2 is usually used for operative office hysteroscopy because it affords a clear view and is quite safe and easy to use.[11] One should use an insufflator designed for hysteroscopy only. The maximum flow rate should be limited to 100 cc/minute, and the maximum pressure should be limited to 100 mm Hg. One can initiate insufflation pressure at 50 mm Hg and increase as needed for adequate visualization. The operator needs to be aware that when working on a patient with patent fallopian tubes, she may experience diaphragmatic irritation and discomfort after insufflation of 600 to 700 cc of CO_2. Patients whose fallopian tubes have been occluded by sterilization or disease can tolerate higher volumes of CO_2. If bleeding occurs, the gynecologist can use the four-toothed tenaculum to close the cervix around the hysteroscope sheath, thus preventing reflux of gas and enhancing intrauterine view.

If blood continues to obscure the view, one can use 32% dextran 70[12] or low-viscosity liquids such as lactated Ringer's or normal saline for visualization, but both have drawbacks for operative hysteroscopy in the office. Thirty-two percent dextran 70 can crystallize and cause locking of hysteroscope valves and instruments. In addition, the amount of 32% dextran 70 should be limited to 300 ml because of the risk of pulmonary edema, blood dyscrasia, and allergic reactions.[13] Low-viscosity liquids, although fine for office diagnostic hysteroscopy, have little place in operative office hysteroscopy because of the large volumes needed and the potential for spilling and resultant messiness.

TECHNIQUE

Operative hysteroscopy can be done any time during the menstrual cycle; however, it is easiest to perform during the early to middle proliferative phase of the cycle. Before any procedure, a thorough history and physical examination are performed along with an assessment of the patient's current medication and general mental status. A recent pap smear, pregnancy test, and hemoglobin and hematocrit levels are prerequisites. Other indicated tests such as cervical cultures for gonorrhea and chlamydia, serum electrolytes, blood sugar, ECG, and chest radiograph may be performed. In my practice, all patients watch a videotape explaining the risks and benefits of this procedure, and an operative permit is signed.

Patients are encouraged to eat a light meal 1 to 2 hours before the procedure. Having something to eat seems to aid in relaxation. A companion must be available to drive the patient home following the examination.

Approximately 30 to 60 minutes before the procedure, the patient is given 550 mm of naproxen sodium or some other nonsteroidal, anti-inflammatory agent. Once in the procedure room, the patient is placed in the lithotomy position, and a pelvic examination is performed. If not done previously, a transvaginal ultrasound may be done to evaluate uterine thickness, screen for intrauterine lesions, and assess the adnexal structures. A 21-gauge needle is inserted in a hand vein if possible, and patency is verified by saline flush. Intravenous diazepam is then slowly injected (up to 5 mg). The intravenous line is flushed again with saline until the patient says all burning is gone, at which point 25 mg of meperidine is administered slowly. Heparin is then instilled in the intravenous line to flush the remaining meperidine and keep the line open in case more analgesia is needed or if an emergency occurs. Alternatively, a continuous IV drip may be used. The medication dosages are adjusted depending on the patient's prior reaction and tolerance. Pulse, respiration, and oxygen saturation are carefully monitored throughout the procedure.

Once the patient is sedated, the vagina is prepped with povidone-iodine. An open-sided speculum is inserted in the vagina, and a paracervical block is given. Usually, 21 ml of a combination of equal amounts of 0.25% bupivacaine and 1% lidocaine hydrochloride is given, which achieves a rapid onset of local anesthesia combined with prolonged activity for those procedures that may take more than an hour. Vasopressin and other vasoactive agents are not used for operative office hysteroscopy. The local anesthetic is given as 10 ml/side and 1 ml in the anterior lip so a tenaculum can be applied. Cervical dilatation is rarely required because the 5-mm sheath can be inserted easily in 90% of procedures.[14]

The cervical canal appears as a dark circle at the 6 o'clock position when using a lens of 25° to 30° (Fig. 10-6). If the angle of view is directed posteriorly, the cervical canal will appear at the 12 o'clock position. Awareness of the direction of view accompanied by careful insertion of the hysteroscope will result in an atraumatic path to the internal os and minimal bleeding. Once the internal os is reached, the operator should pause and let the distention medium open the os to allow careful entry into the uterine cavity (Fig. 10-7).

An overall view of the uterine cavity should be made at this time, noting the endometrial appearance, the cavity's general shape, and the presence of any foreign bodies, synechiae, polyps, leiomyomas, septa, unusual lumps, bumps, or discoloration. The hysteroscope is advanced slowly and rotated clockwise and counterclockwise to view the left and right cornua and tubal ostia. Once the entire uterine cavity has been examined, the hysteroscope is removed slowly, and the cervical canal is re-examined; it usually can be seen better when the scope is being withdrawn rather than when it is being inserted.

If abnormal uterine bleeding is the hysteroscopic indication and no lesion is seen in the uterine cavity, a suction curettage is performed using a 5-, 6-, or 7-mm curette. After

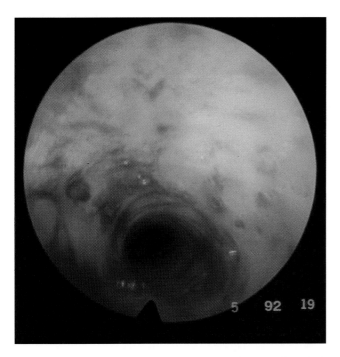

Fig. 10-6. Cervical canal appearing as dark circle at 6 o'clock position.

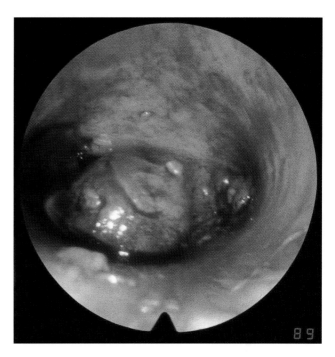

Fig. 10-8. Polyp found in uterine cavity obscured by blood after suction curettage.

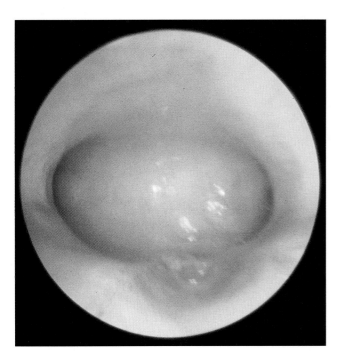

Fig. 10-7. View of uterine cavity from internal cervical os.

curettage, the hysteroscope is reinserted because a polyp or leiomyoma may be exposed after the removal of blood or surface endometrium[8] (Fig. 10-8). If there is any surface irregularity or discoloration, the operating hysteroscope should be inserted before curettage, and directed biopsy of the suspicious area should be performed with a flexible or semirigid biopsy forceps. This directed biopsy will give a more accurate diagnosis than will a curettage.[4,15] Cervical dilatation is rarely needed, because the diagnostic scope can be inserted 90% of the time without it and 90% of the time will dilate the canal sufficiently to allow a 7-mm operative sheath to be inserted anyway. If dilatation is necessary, it should be performed gently, avoiding overextension, because operative office hysteroscopy is best performed with a tight cervical seal around the hysteroscope sheath. If the cervix is overdistended or patulous, the four-toothed cervical-sealing tenaculum can be used to grasp the cervical lips and compress them around the hysteroscope sheath to prevent reflux of the distention medium.

SUBMUCOUS LEIOMYOMA

Myomectomy, if done in the office, is one of the most satisfying operations for both the patient and the gynecologist. Myomas that are smaller than 2 cm and pedunculated are usually removed with ease. One grasps the myoma with the myoma grasper or a pituitary rongeur, twists the leiomyoma free from its attachment to the myometrium, and pulls it out of the uterine cavity (Fig. 10-9).[16] This procedure may be done either under direct vision or blindly after first visualizing the leiomyoma to evaluate its depth and location in the uterine cavity. Following adequate dilatation, the myoma grasper is inserted through the cervical canal with its jaws closed. Once inside the uterine cavity, the jaws are opened, and the myoma is grasped. When the lesion has been removed, the hysteroscope must be reinserted to confirm that removal has been complete. Any residual small fragments can be removed with a grasping forceps through the operat-

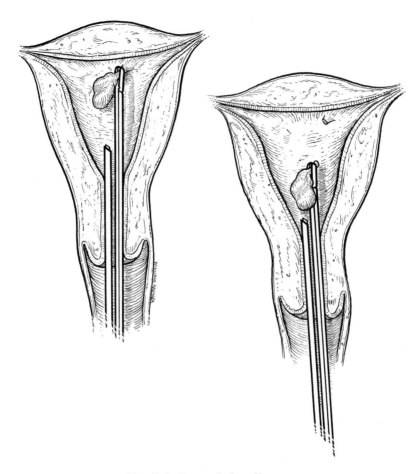

Fig. 10-9. Removal of small myoma.

ing hysteroscope. To grasp larger fragments under direct vision, the pituitary rongeur may be inserted alongside the hysteroscope (usually the diagnostic sheath). With increasing skill, the surgeon can remove pedunculated leiomyomas as large as 4 cm (Fig. 10-10). If the cervix is overdilated to allow insertion of a diagnostic hysteroscope and myoma grasper or pituitary rongeur for direct visualization of the myoma, the cervical canal can be sealed to prevent CO_2 leakage by applying the four-toothed cervical-sealing tenaculum. Myomas that are sessile and 2 cm or less in diameter but at least 50% intrauterine can be removed by carefully incising the capsule with flexible or semirigid scissors. Preoperative transvaginal ultrasound is beneficial in revealing the myometrial thickness distal to the base of the leiomyoma. The leiomyoma is then excised from its bed in much the same manner as that used for a submucous leiomyoma at laparoscopy or laparotomy. As the myoma is freed up, it will increasingly protrude into the uterine cavity until it can be treated in the same manner as a pedunculated leiomyoma. Bleeding that requires the procedure to be stopped is rare, although the surgeon must be careful to avoid incising obvious vessels.

If a leiomyoma is 1 cm in diameter, it can usually be removed hysteroscopically even if only a small portion is seen

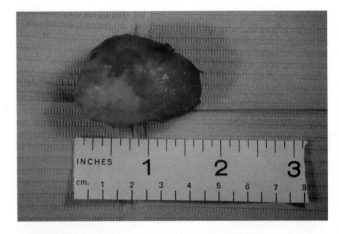

Fig. 10-10. Large pedunculated leiomyoma removed in operative office hysteroscopy.

protruding into the uterine cavity. If a pituitary rongeur can grasp it, the myoma can usually be extracted intact just as a dentist would extract a tooth. If most of the 1-cm leiomyoma is intramural, the capsule can be incised as described above and, as it protrudes into the uterine cavity, grasped and extracted intact (Fig. 10-11).

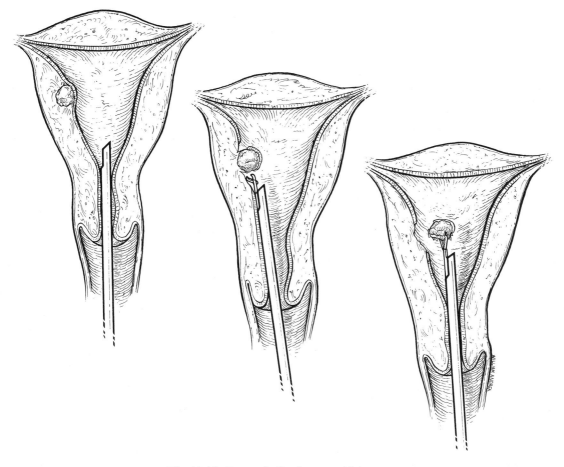

Fig. 10-11. Removal of an intramural leiomyoma.

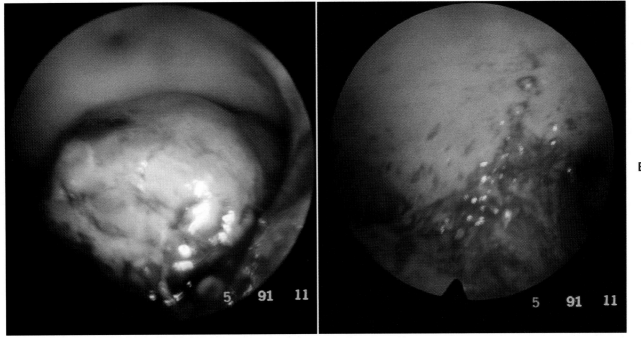

Fig. 10-12. A, Endometrial polyp occupying most of right cornu. **B,** View of the uterine cavity 1 month postoperatively.

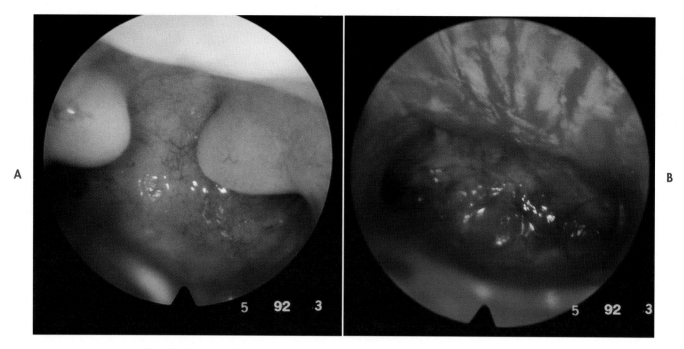

Fig. 10-13. **A,** Multiple endometrial polyps. **B,** Uterine cavity after suction curettage.

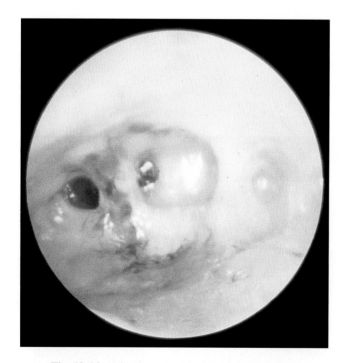

Fig. 10-14. Adhesion with a mainly central location.

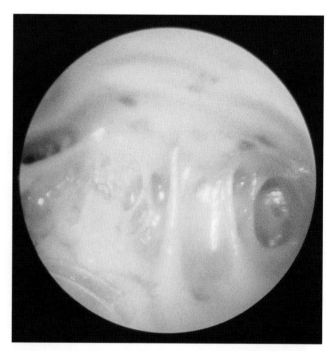

Fig. 10-15. Diffuse, thick adhesions.

ENDOMETRIAL POLYPS

Any size of pedunculated endometrial polyp can be removed in the office. The polyp is grasped or incised at its base and separated from the uterine wall. Because polyps are generally softer than leiomyomas, they can be easily removed from the uterine cavity with less need for cervical dilatation than myomas. Large polyps can be morcellated

with the primary rongeur or myoma grasper, although they may also be removed intact, as is the case with small polyps. (Fig. 10-12). Sometimes multiple small polyps are present in the uterine cavity. Rather than removing each one individually, the optimal approach is suction curettage followed by re-examination with the hysteroscope (Fig. 10-13). Broad-based sessile polyps do not lend themselves to com-

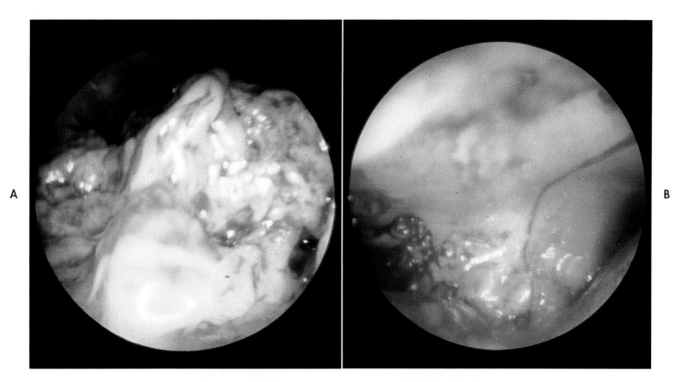

Fig. 10-16. A, Retained products of conception following mid-trimester abortion and two D&Cs. **B,** Uterine cavity 1 month following operative office hysteroscopy.

plete removal in the office and may require follow-up treatment in the operating room using a laser or resectoscope.

INTRAUTERINE ADHESIONS

Intrauterine adhesions that are centrally located may be easily divided in the office with flexible or semirigid scissors. In fact, any adhesions that can be seen around may be divided in the office (Fig. 10-14). However, diffuse adhesions are best divided in an operating room under laparoscopic guidance, because the risk of perforation is higher (Fig. 10-15). Lateral adhesions also are often best approached in the operating room because the direction of incision is often confusing, and laparoscopy can help direct the procedure or reveal a small perforation. Ultrasound to assess uterine wall thickness may allow a more aggressive approach in the office. Once adhesions have been divided, a follow-up diagnostic hysteroscopy should be done in the office.

Hysteroscopic lysis of adhesions is a meticulous process that should not be hurried, especially when performed in the office. It is acceptable to stop the surgery before completion if bleeding begins to obscure vision or if the patient becomes uncomfortable secondary to intraperitoneal accumulation of CO_2. A hysterosalpingogram should always be done to guide the surgical pathway before lysing intrauterine adhesions.

LOST INTRAUTERINE DEVICE

One of the easiest operative office hysteroscopic procedures is removal of a lost IUD. The first step in evaluating the patient without a visible IUD string is ultrasonography, which will usually reveal the device's intrauterine or extrauterine location.[17] After ultrasound confirms the intrauterine location, hysteroscopy proceeds as described in the basic technique. First the 5-mm diagnostic sheath with 4-mm telescope is inserted to confirm the intrauterine location of the IUD. At this point, if the cervix is easily traversed, a pituitary rongeur is inserted alongside the hysteroscope, and the IUD is grasped and removed under direct vision. Another approach is to remove the diagnostic sheath and insert an operating hysteroscope. Once the IUD string is seen, a flexible or semirigid grasper is inserted through the operating channel, and the string is grasped and delivered into the vagina. Then a stronger grasper takes hold of the IUD string and removes the device from the uterine cavity. If partial perforation is documented, the procedure shifts to the operating room for laparoscopic guidance.

RETAINED PRODUCTS OF CONCEPTION

Fragments of placenta sometimes remain inside the uterus after an abortion or delivery. These retained fragments may result in persistent bleeding episodes that require repeat curettage. At some point a hysteroscopic examination becomes more beneficial than continued blind curettage (Fig. 10-16, A) and can easily be done in an office setting. Once the retained products are visualized, they can be removed in much the same manner as a leiomyoma or polyp. The uterine cavity should be examined 1 month after removal of the retained products to ensure that synechiae have

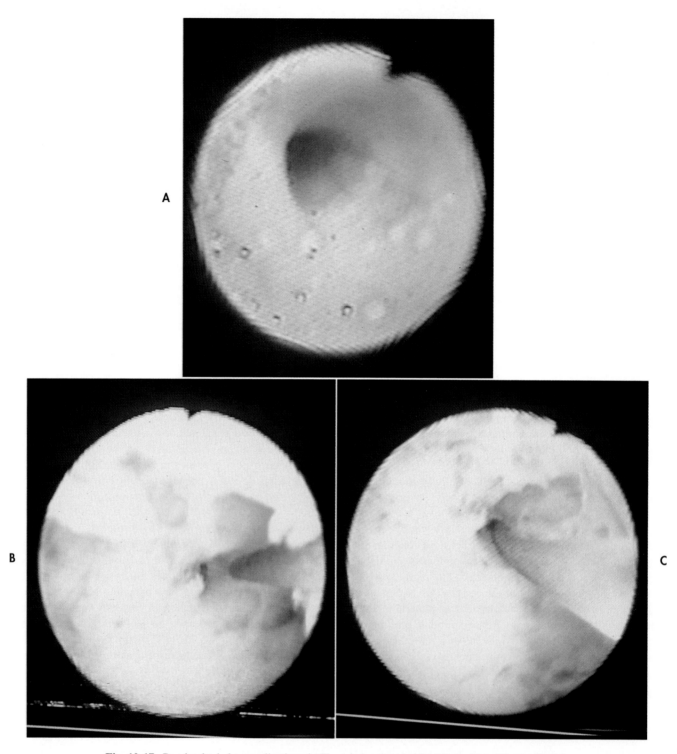

Fig. 10-17. Proximal tubal recanalization. **A,** The tubal ostium is identified with a 4.9-mm flexible hysteroscope (Olympus HYF-1T), using normal saline for uterine distention. **B,** A 0.035-inch angled-tip, Teflon-coated guidewire (Meditech, Boston Scientific Corp., Watertown, Mass) is placed down the 2.2-mm working channel and directed into the tubal ostium. **C,** The guidewire is advanced through the proximal tubal obstruction and into the ampulla of the fallopian tube.

not formed or, if they have, that they are lysed in the early stage (Fig. 10-16, *B*).

FALLOPIAN TUBE CANNULATION

Proximal tubal obstruction is present in up to 10% of infertile women. Daniell and Miller[18] first reported on a hysteroscopic correction of cornual occlusion in 1987, and since that time many office tubal recanalizations have been performed. Before the gynecologist performs office tubal recanalization, the patient will have had at least two hysterosalpingograms or a hysterosalpingogram and chromopertubation at laparoscopy to confirm the diagnosis of proximal tubal obstruction. On the evening before and the morning of the procedure the patient is given 100 mg of doxycycline by mouth. A 4.9-mm flexible hysteroscope is then placed within the cervix and advanced under direct visualization using either CO_2 or normal saline for uterine distention. No cervical dilatation or paracervical anesthesia is necessary in 75% of patients. The flexible hysteroscope has a 2.2-mm working channel, which will allow the passage of a 0.035-inch plastic-coated glidewire.* Once the tip of the flexible scope is placed near the tubal ostium, the guidewire is advanced into the fallopian tube (Fig. 10-17). If the guidewire is within the interstitium of the fallopian tube and cannot be advanced, then it is likely the tube is fibrosed and not blocked with a plug of cellular debris.[19] At this point the procedure should be abandoned and the patient referred for resection and reanastomosis or IVF. Using this technique, we have been able to recannulate at least one tube in 87% of patients on whom we have attempted the procedure. After 6 months, at least one fallopian tube has remained open in 60% of patients.

Transcervical catheterization of the fallopian tube without falloposcopy can also be done under fluoroscopic guidance and thus is not applicable to an office setting.[20] Transvaginal sonography has allowed tubal evaluation, but the transvaginal probe precludes concomitant use of the hysteroscope.[20]

Cannulation has been used experimentally for transcervical tubal sterilization. The two most effective sterilization methods used via cannula were electrocoagulation of the intramural portion of the fallopian tube[22] and instillation of silicone plugs.[23,24] Both procedures achieved up to 90% success, each with nearly 100% occlusion of tubes bilaterally. However, both procedures had inherent problems and never received FDA clearance for marketing in the United States. Following initial studies with electrocoagulation, results of a multicenter collaborative study showed not only less than 60% bilateral tubal occlusion but also that electrocoagulation was associated with major complications, including tubal and cornual ectopic pregnancies, bowel injuries, peritonitis, and even one death.[25]

Between 1978 and 1984 at 30 centers for investigation, occlusion of the fallopian tubes with silicone plugs was very successful, with minimal complications in more than 2000 women. Long-term adverse effects have been minimal; however, carcinoma occurred in one group of laboratory animals, and FDA clearance has never been given in the United States although the procedure is being carried out in the Netherlands.[26]

I mainly use hysteroscopic tubal catheterization today to divide cornual and very proximal tubal adhesions. Essentially any SFR catheter can be inserted into the proximal ostia to dilate the opening and divide synechiae in the most proximal portion of the tube. At this point, low-viscosity fluids can be instilled through the cannula and, if easily passed, one can assume the tube is open. Similarly, one can instill CO_2 through the cannula and if the patient experiences shoulder pain, it can be assumed the tube is open. Most successful tubal cannulation for proximal occlusion should be performed under fluoroscopic guidance or with falloposcopy, which is discussed in Chapter 13.

POSTOPERATIVE CARE

At the end of the procedure, the patient is given written instructions and advised to avoid intercourse and alcohol for 48 hours. The instructions (see adjacent box) advise the patient to call the physician if she has severe pain, fever greater than 101° F, or excessive bleeding. Usually the patient is seen in 1 week for a follow-up examination and discussion of the pathology report. A nonsteroidal, antiinflammatory agent is given for the mild cramps that occasionally follow the procedure.

Postoperative instructions for panoramic hysteroscopy and/or dilatation and curettage

Rest this evening.

Avoid alcoholic beverages for 48 hours.

Avoid intercourse for 48 hours.

Make an appointment to be seen in my office in one week to discuss the pathology report and plan for future treatments if necessary.

Notify me if any of the following occurs:
Fever above 101° F
Severe pains
Bleeding that requires more pads than a normal period

You should expect some drainage and some bleeding that may continue for several days or even up until your next period

Your next period may be very light or may be heavy. Do not be alarmed by either change.

If you need to notify me of any problems after office hours, please call my medical exchange at _____.

---

*Glidewire, Terumo, Inc, Watertown, Mass.

_____	$50.00	Hysteroscopy pack (sterile speculum, tenaculum, ring forceps, uterine sound, hysteroscope, sheaths)
_____	35.00	Surgical pack (sterile speculum, tenaculum, ring forceps)
_____	5.00	Sterile drapes
_____	2.00	Sterile gloves
_____	2.00	Sterile gauze
_____	1.00	Cotton balls
_____	2.00	Sterile cotton-tipped applicators
_____	3.00	3-ml syringe
_____	1.00	10-ml syringe
_____	2.00	20-ml syringe
_____	2.00	30-ml syringe
_____	2.00	60-ml syringe
_____	5.00	Spinal needle
_____	1.00	20g 1½-inch needle
_____	1.00	27g ½-inch needle
_____	1.00	Saline
_____	1.00	Acetic acid
_____	1.00	Lugol's solution
_____	2.00	Monsel's solution
_____	1.00	Betadine solution
_____	2.00	Bupivacaine 0.25%
_____	2.00	Lidocaine 1%
_____	2.00	Demerol
_____	5.00	Versed
_____	4.00	Valium
_____	2.00	Anaprox
_____	2.00	Cidex
_____	35.00	Hyskon
_____	2.00	Plastic tube for suction
_____	100.00	Avitene
_____	5.00	CO_2 & CO_2 tube
_____	5.00	Smoke evacuator filter
_____	3.00	Surgical masks
_____	20.00	Uterine tissue traps
_____	15.00	Uterine exploratory curette
_____	1.00	Bacteriostatic NaCl
_____	1.00	Heparin solution
_____	3.00	Butterfly infusion set
_____	8.00	Pitressin solution
_____	8.00	Suture
_____	30.00	Electrical generator
_____	5.00	Electrical loop
_____	2.00	Examination gloves
_____	4.00	Barrier gown
_____	1.00	Shoe covers
_____	1.00	Surgical caps

PATIENT: _____

SURGICAL PROCEDURE: _____

DATE: _____

PATIENT NUMBER _____

TOTAL _____

REIMBURSEMENT

Operative office hysteroscopy should be reimbursed at the same level as operative hysteroscopy in an operating room. In addition, the gynecologist who does office hysteroscopy and administers and monitors anesthesia should be paid for these services, as well as for supplies used during the procedure. The charges for supplies used in the office are much lower than the charges for supplies used in an operating room of a hospital or outpatient surgery center. Many third-party payers and managed care plans realize the savings and are willing to reimburse the physician for these additional supply expenses. However, some third-party payers do not reimburse for supplies used in the office or anesthesia given by the operating surgeon. This practice is one of the factors in the rise of health care costs. All supplies used during a procedure are itemized and submitted separately so it is clear to the insurance company what items have been used and what reimbursement is sought. An example of an itemized supply list used in my office practice is shown in the box.

CONCLUSION

Just as diagnostic hysteroscopy has become an office procedure, operative hysteroscopy can be performed in the office quite easily. One needs the proper equipment, patient selection, and experience to perform extensive operative office hysteroscopy. The ability to do diagnostic and operative hysteroscopy at the same time results in a substantial savings of both cost and time for the patient and physician.

One final note: in today's climate of concern over AIDS transmission, office surgeries require strict adherence to OSHA guidelines. This includes surgical attire (gown, gloves, mask, head cover, and shoe covers) and protective eye wear for the operating surgeon and assistants.

REFERENCES

1. Goldrath MH, Sherman AL: Office hysteroscopy and suction curettage: can we eliminate the hospital diagnostic dilatation & curettage? _Am J Obstet Gynecol_ 152:220, 1984.
2. Gimpelson RJ: Office hysteroscopy indications and limitations, _The female patient_ 14:14, 1989.
3. Gimpelson RJ: Office hysteroscopy, _Clin Obstet Gynecol_ 35:2, April-June 1992.
4. Gimpelson RJ, Rappold HO: A comparative study between panoramic hysteroscopy with direct biopsies and dilatation and curettage, _Am J Obstet Gynecol_ 158:489, 1988.
5. Valle RF, Sciarra JJ: Current status of hysteroscopy in gynecologic practice, _Fertil Steril_ 32:619, 1979.
6. Sciarra JJ, Valle RF: A clinical experience with 320 patients, _Am J Obstet Gynecol_ 127:340, 1977.
7. Hamou J, Salat-Baroux J: Advanced hysteroscopy and micro-hysteroscopy: our experience with 1000 patients. In Siegler AM, Lindemann HJ, Eds: _Hysteroscopy: principles and practice_, Philadelphia, 1984, JB Lippincott.
8. Gimpelson RJ, Hill J: Suction curettage with a tissue trap compared with sharp curettage for tissue sampling, _J Reprod Med_ 36:7, 1991.

9. Siegler AM et al: Instruments. In Siegler AM, Ed: *Therapeutic hysteroscopy: indications and techniques,* St. Louis, 1990, Mosby.

10. Gimpelson RJ: Preventing cervical reflux of the distention media during panoramic hysteroscopy, *J Reprod Med* 31:7, 1986.

11. Lindemann HJ, Mohr JW: CO_2 hysteroscopy: diagnosis and treatment, *Am J Obstet Gynecol* 124:129, 1976.

12. Edstrom K, Fernstrom I: The diagnostic possibilities of a modified hysteroscopic technique, *Acta Obstet Gynecol Scand* 49:327, 1970.

13. Ahmed N et al: Anaphylactic reaction because of intrauterine 32% dextran-70 instillation, *Fertil Steril* 55:1014, 1991.

14. Gimpelson RJ: Experience with the Autonom 4992 self-contained panoramic hysteroscope, *J Reprod Med* 33:11, 1988.

15. Brooks PG, Serden SP: Hysteroscopic findings after unsuccessful dilatation and curettage for abnormal bleeding, *Am J Obstet Gynecol* 158:1354, 1988.

16. Goldrath MH: Vaginal removal of the pedunculated submucous myoma: the use of laminaria, *Obstet Gynecol* 70:670, 1987.

17. Callen PW, Fily RA, Munyer TP: Intrauterine contraceptive devices: evaluation by sonography, *AJR* 135:797, 1980.

18. Daniell JF, Miller W: Hysteroscopic correction of cornual occlusion with resultant term pregnancy, *Fertil Steril* 48:490, 1987.

19. Sulak PJ et al: Histology of proximal tubal occlusion, *Fertil Steril* 48:437, 1987.

20. Risquez F, Confino E: Transcervical tubal cannulation: past, present and future, *Fertil Steril* 60:211, 1993.

21. Tufeci EC et al: Evaluation of tubal patency by transvaginal sonosalpingography, *Fertil Steril* 57:336, 1992.

22. Quinones-Guerro R, Aznar-Ramos R, Duran HA: Tubal electrocauterization under hysteroscopic control, *Contraception* 7:195, 1973.

23. Houk RM, Cooper JM, Rigberg HS: Hysteroscopic tubal occlusion with formed-in-place silicone plugs: clinical review, *Obstet Gynecol* 62:587, 1983.

24. Reed TP, Erb R: Hysteroscopic tubal occlusion with silicone rubber, *Obstet Gynecol* 61:388, 1983.

25. Cooper JM: Hysteroscopic sterilization, *Clin Obstet Gynecol* 35:282, 1991.

26. Discussions with Ovabloc Inc, Stamford, Conn. (Unpublished data.)

Chapter 11

OFFICE HYSTEROSCOPY: COMPLICATIONS AND MANAGEMENT

Kees Wamsteker

Apart from diagnostic procedures, office hysteroscopy may include minor intrauterine interventions such as endometrial biopsies, polypectomies, minor adhesiolysis, and IUD removal. Because of the limited operative facilities and time constraints of a busy practice, the majority of office hysteroscopy cases will be purely diagnostic, with an occasional diagnostic biopsy. In some cases, however, the "office" procedures will be performed in an ambulatory unit with more facilities, equipment, and specialized personnel, which enables minor intrauterine surgical interventions to be done. This chapter on complications and their management during office hysteroscopy will therefore include those that occur during diagnostic and minor endosurgical procedures, as well as in connection with the application of local anesthesia.

With proper techniques and adequate experience, complications in office hysteroscopy will be extremely rare. The possible complications can be divided into four subgroups: those arising from trauma, from uterine distention, from impaired visualization, or from local anesthetics. These subgroups will be discussed in succession.

TRAUMATIC COMPLICATIONS

Traumatic complications during office hysteroscopy generally arise from improper instrument management. Most frequently they occur not during the hysteroscopic procedure itself but during blind sounding of the uterus or dilatation of the internal cervical os in sharply anteverted or retroverted uteri before the actual hysteroscopic procedure. This traumatic damage can cause bleeding and lead to a false route, which may result in a uterine perforation directly or during the following hysteroscopy. A false route is most likely to occur at the area just before the internal cervical os or at the fundus of the uterine cavity.

In case of a very tight internal os, the tenaculum can tear the cervix during dilatation, creating significant bleeding if the attachment of the tenaculum to the cervix is not firm enough. In diagnostic procedures using hysteroscopes that are 5 mm or less in diameter, little to no dilatation will be necessary, and this complication is unusual.

During the hysteroscopic procedure itself, uterine perforation is extremely rare and should not occur. Generally it will result from using improper technique and will be caused mostly by proceeding forward with the hysteroscope without adequate distention and panoramic view or with otherwise impaired visualization.

Hysteroscopy should be performed as much as possible with a no-touch technique. A complete no-touch procedure is not possible, but touching the walls of the endocervix and the uterine cavity should be avoided as much as possible to prevent traumatic complications. To this purpose the hysteroscope should always be inserted under visual control with adequate distention, starting in the endocervix.

The incidence of traumatic complications during office hysteroscopy is not known. In the majority of cases, complications will occur because of lack of experience in the learning phase. In experienced hands, they almost always occur because of a pathologic condition, such as intracervical or intracavitary adhesions.

With D&C procedures the estimated incidence of uterine perforations is 6 to 13 per 1000.[1] With hysteroscopy the incidence will be significantly lower, because the uterus should not be blindly sounded before the procedure; also the required dilatation of the internal cervical os is less, and the hysteroscopy is performed under visual control. Lindemann[2] and Lindemann and Mohr[3] reported 6 perforations in 5220 procedures. Barrôcco et al,[4] Raju and Taylor,[5] De Jong et al,[6] and Hill et al[7] reported no complications in outpatient hysteroscopy in 998 cases.

Prevention of traumatic complications

A very important step in preventing traumatic complications is the bimanual vaginal examination that occurs immediately before the procedure. The exact position of the uterus should be determined and kept in mind during insertion of the hysteroscope and/or dilatation of the internal cervical canal.[8]

There is no indication to sound the uterus before the hysteroscopic procedure. When the internal cervical os has to be dilated, this should be performed very gently with blunt,

half-sized Hegar dilators. The elastic, circular structure of the internal cervical os should be felt to give way smoothly, and the dilator must not be inserted farther than the internal os itself. The dilatation should never be performed forcefully. In case the resistance seems to be greater than normal, prior endocervical hysteroscopic inspection is mandatory to rule out any pathology or an abnormally located internal os. In the majority of cases, the hysteroscope can be inserted under direct visual control without prior dilatation of the internal os.

With rigid instruments, the hysteroscope must be inserted in a more upward direction ("take-off" position) when there is sharp anteflexion of the uterus and in a more downward position ("landing" position) when there is a retroverted uterus. The hysteroscope is placed into the endocervix (Fig. 11-1, *A*), and the endocervical canal is visualized. If the hysteroscope has a 30° foreoblique viewing angle, it may need to be moved and/or rotated upward, downward, or laterally

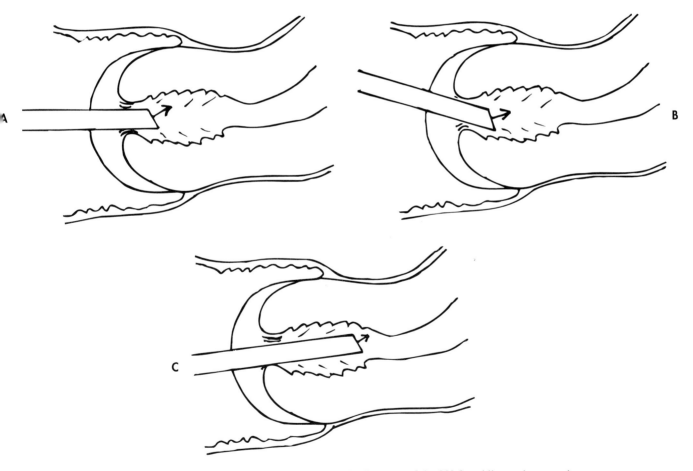

Fig. 11-1. A, Hysteroscope tip in distal endocervix. Because of the 30° foreoblique telescope, the complete endocervix and internal os may not yet be visualized (*arrow* indicates viewing direction). **B,** Upward movement of the ocular end of the hysteroscope enables visualization of the complete endocervix and internal os. **C,** To enable atraumatic passage of the internal os in an anteverted uterus, the hysteroscope has to be brought in a more or less "take-off" position; because of the 30° foreoblique telescope, mainly the anterior wall of the endocervix and internal os will be seen. The posterior wall should not be visible in the image. The instrument used is a rigid, single-flow 4- or 5-mm diagnostic hysteroscope (Olympus).

until the full length of the endocervical canal with the internal os is visualized (Fig. 11-1, *B*).

Visualization of the endocervix with CO_2 distention and a single-channel hysteroscope (Fig. 11-2) may be difficult because of the cervical mucus. For this reason we prefer continuous-flow (double-channel) hysteroscopes (Fig. 11-3) with low-viscosity fluids[9] even though the diameter of these instruments is slightly increased (5.5 mm) compared with single-channel hysteroscopes (3.6 to 5 mm). The advantage of the continuous-flow hysteroscope is the excellent visualization obtained in this area during the introduction of the instrument. This benefit is of utmost importance, especially for physicians who are learning the procedure.

When resistance to the hysteroscope at the internal os is too high for a smooth, atraumatic insertion and the internal cervical os is maximally dilated (up to the diameter of the hysteroscope), local anesthesia may be required. This situation is more likely to occur in nulliparous or postmenopausal women.[8]

As mentioned, the hysteroscope should always pass the internal cervical os under direct visual control. In doing so, one must realize that the tip of the hysteroscope has a blunt angle of 150° and a sharp angle of 30°. If the sharp angle touches the tissue, it will scrape off mucosa; by contrast, the blunt angle will slide more smoothly over the tissue. Passing through the internal cervical os, the hysteroscope tip should be advanced with the blunt angle over the anterior wall, thus preventing the sharp angle from touching the posterior wall (Fig. 11-1, *C*). Using this technique, only the upper part of the internal cervical os itself will be seen in the lower part of the image. After entering the uterine cavity, the hysteroscope should be moved upward to achieve a full panoramic view. The tip of the hysteroscope should not touch the endometrium, and the hysteroscope should not be advanced without adequate distention and visualization. If the hysteroscope is pushed forward while touching the endometrium, a piece of the mucosa will be scraped off and will impair visualization.

With CO_2 distention, some mucus and blood in the uterine cavity can hamper visualization. In those cases, the hysteroscope should never be advanced but should be withdrawn slightly until visualization is restored. In case of persistent impaired visualization, it is much safer to change to noncontinuous- or continuous-flow hysteroscopy with liquid distention. This strategy will immediately clear the uterine cavity and restore visualization.

Finally, the hysteroscopic procedure should always be performed in the early proliferative phase of the menstrual cycle immediately following the cessation of menses, or the patient should be taking oral contraceptives or other medication to flatten the endometrium. The thick, late proliferative and secretory endometrium can hide pathology and endometrial fragments that will easily be detached from their base by the tip of the hysteroscope.

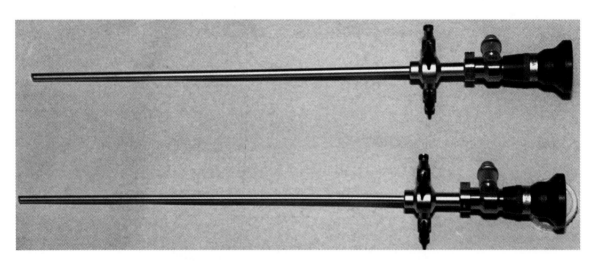

Fig. 11-2. Rigid, single-flow 4- or 5-mm diagnostic hysteroscope (Olympus).

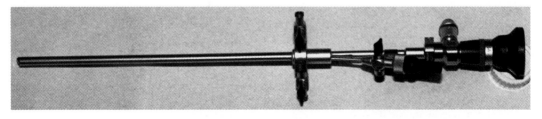

Fig. 11-3. Rigid, continuous-flow 5.5-mm diagnostic hysteroscope (Olympus).

Conditions predisposing to uterine perforation

A uterus in a sharp anteverted or retroverted position predisposes to the formation of a false route if the aforementioned precautions are not taken into account. In addition, pathologic conditions can predispose to uterine perforation. For example, adhesions in the endocervix or in the uterine cavity can lead to a false route, especially in the case of prior blunt attempts to lyse them. Adhesions should always be dissolved very carefully under visual control. The hysteroscope should not be used to lyse adhesions if at least one of the tubal ostia is not visible. In this condition, hysteroscopic synechiolysis must be performed under general anesthesia with laparoscopic control. Firm adhesions should always be dissected with scissors and forceps.[10]

Submucous or intramural myomata in the lower part of the uterus can distort the endocervix, displacing the cervical canal and isthmic channel. Under visual control, the hysteroscope can be safely manipulated around these distortions.

Management of traumatic complications

Should a severe laceration of the ectocervix occur during removal of the tenaculum, it must be closed with one or two stitches. The repair is usually done with 0 chromic suture.

There have been no reported cases of uterine perforation with a flexible hysteroscope. Perforation of the fundal area of the uterus with a rigid diagnostic hysteroscope will generally not lead to serious sequelae. A small perforation will almost never result in severe intra-abdominal bleeding and will close almost immediately after withdrawal of the hysteroscope. However, the patient must be observed for several hours, and a short course of antibiotics may be considered. If operating instruments have been used through the perforated opening before the perforation was noticed, intestinal damage may have occurred, which could lead to serious complications. In those cases, which should never happen with adequate technique, the patient must be observed for at least 24 hours. If any doubt exists as to whether real intestinal damage has occurred, a laparoscopy should be performed.

If a perforation occurs in the lateral sidewalls of the uterus and reaches into the parametrium, major vessels may be damaged, and a laparoscopy must be performed immediately or the patient must be observed for at least 24 hours. Likewise, possible perforation of the bladder requires immediate confirmation and repair. These types of perforations, however, will be extremely rare during diagostic hysteroscopy in which proper technique is used.

Minor bleeding or detachment of the mucosa of the endocervix or the uterus needs no further treatment.

COMPLICATIONS FROM DISTENTION MEDIA

The distention media for hysteroscopy have been dealt with extensively in Chapter 6. Some aspects related to complications will be discussed briefly in this chapter.

Originally different distention media were used for diagnostic hysteroscopy and hysteroscopic endosurgery. Diagnostic hysteroscopy was generally performed with non-continuous-flow hysteroscopes using CO_2 or high-viscosity dextran 70 solution (Hyskon) for distention. For hysteroscopic endosurgery, continuous-flow operating hysteroscopes or resectoscopes are used with pressurized, low-viscosity fluids. Recently, continuous-flow hysteroscopes have also been developed for diagnostic purposes, and this method is being applied increasingly. Continuous-flow diagnostic hysteroscopy providing superior clarity in visualizing the endocervical canal and uterine cavity will eventually replace CO_2 and dextran in diagnostic hysteroscopy. Possible complications from the distention media will be discussed in relation to the different media.

CO_2

Originally CO_2 insufflation for hysteroscopy resulted in serious complications caused by cardiac CO_2 embolism. Extensive animal studies by Lindemann et al[11] have defined safety limits for the flow and pressure of CO_2 insufflation for hysteroscopy. As long as the flow does not exceed 100 cc/minute, with a maximum insufflation pressure of 150 mm Hg (safety range up to 200 mm Hg), there is no risk from CO_2 intravasation. Since these studies were published, specific hysteroscopic insufflators have been developed that restrict the flow and insufflation pressure according to established safety limits. No other insufflation equipment should ever be used.

Brundin and Thomassen[12] and Rythen-Alder et al[13] have reported a 50% incidence in mill-wheel murmur sounds at precordial auscultation and gas embolism detected by echocardiography performed during CO_2 hysteroscopy, even with CO_2 flow and pressure within the safety limits. However, these cases did not result in clinical complications. The quantity of cardiac embolization appeared to be positively related with the insufflation pressure, as well as with intrauterine manipulation. From these data, one can conclude that during diagnostic hysteroscopy with CO_2 distention, the intrauterine pressure should be kept as low as possible.

If a procedure with CO_2 distention is somewhat more extended in combination with patent tubes, the patient may get shoulder pain caused by intra-abdominal CO_2.

Brooks (1995 personal communication) reported three cases of possible air embolism during CO_2 hysteroscopy in patients placed in the Trendelenburg position. It was hypothesized that negative pressure in ruptured uterine veins caused the problem. It may therefore be advisable to avoid a steep Trendelenburg position in hysteroscopy with gas distention.

As long as the safety limitations for insufflation flow rates and pressures are followed, hysteroscopy with CO_2 distention is a safe procedure.

Dextran solutions

In the past, highly viscous dextran solutions were used for diagnostic hysteroscopy. The solution most commonly used was a 32% dextran 70 solution in 10% dextrose, which is available as Hyskon. Because it is rather difficult to inject through a single-flow diagnostic hysteroscope, we preferred diluting the Hyskon solution for diagnostic procedures with 10 ml of saline in 100 ml Hyskon. Intravasation of Hyskon in endosurgical procedures can result in circulatory fluid overload and pulmonary edema. Because of its hyperosmolarity, absorption of 100 ml of Hyskon will expand the circulating volume by about 860 ml.[14] In diagnostic procedures the risk for a significant amount of intravasation of the highly viscous dextran solution is negligible because no myometrial vessels are opened and the procedures are brief. Generally not more than 60 to 80 ml will be used, most of which will flow out through the cervix.

Dextran also can cause anaphylactic reactions after intravasation or intraperitoneal application. Borton et al[15] estimated this reaction to occur in approximately 1 in 10,000 cases. It can vary from a minor skin rash to serious anaphylactic shock. Other reactions can include bronchospasm and muscular cramps. The allergic reaction is not dependent on the amount of dextran given and often occurs early in the infusion process. Prior exposure to dextran is not necessary to develop these reactions.[14] The anaphylactic reaction can be almost completely prevented, via hapten inhibition, by preadministering small amounts of intravenous dextran just before the procedure.[16]

When one suspects an allergic reaction, the dextran injection should be terminated immediately, and the patient must get intravenous fluids and oxygen. Further therapy consists of prednisolone sodium phosphate 25 mg IV and, in case of bradycardia, 0.5 mg atropine IM. If hypotension develops, adrenaline 0.5 ml (1:1000) IM should be administered. Persistent bronchospasm should be controlled with aminophylline 240 mg given slowly IV.

Because allergic reactions to Hyskon are very rare in diagnostic hysteroscopy, the medium is considered to be relatively safe for uterine distention in hysteroscopy. However, equipment and medication for emergency treatment of anaphylactic reactions should be available in the procedure room.[17]

Another disadvantage of Hyskon is that it caramelizes upon drying. This property results in malfunction of the hysteroscopic equipment. The moving parts, such as stopcocks and forceps, will freeze. To prevent this caramelization, all exposed equipment must be flushed and thoroughly cleaned in warm water and with a neutral detergent immediately after the procedure.

Low-viscosity fluids

Low-viscosity fluids, originally used exclusively in hysteroscopic endosurgical procedures, are now being used increasingly for diagnostic procedures with continuous-flow and noncontinuous-flow hysteroscopes. The liquids used are 3% sorbitol, 1.5% glycine, 5% dextrose, lactated Ringer's solution, and saline. Because D_5LR and saline are not suit-

able for high-frequency electrosurgery, they should not be used for resectoscopy. Further specific advantages and disadvantages of these different liquid media were discussed in Chapter 6. The most important complication of using low-viscosity fluids, especially if they are applied with more than just hydrostatic pressure, is excessive intravasation, which may result in overfilling the circulation, electrolyte disturbances, and pulmonary edema. The high level of intravasation will occur almost only in surgical procedures. In diagnostic procedures, the liquids can be administered with a hydrostatic pressure of 1 meter. However, in case of minor diagnostic intrauterine procedures, the use of additional pressure is recommended. The required amount of liquid for a reliable diagnostic procedure will seldom be more than 1 L, most of which will be re-collected from the outflow channel. The most important parameter for the intravasation of liquid is "fluid loss," the difference between infused and regained fluids. The regained fluid should include both the fluid from the outflow channel and the fluid flushing out from the vagina. The fluid must be collected in a calibrated bottle to accurately tally the total amount of loss (Fig. 11-4).

Because the risk of excessive intravasation in diagnostic procedures is almost nonexistent, low-viscosity fluids with continuous-flow instruments have the least risk for complications in diagnostic office procedures.

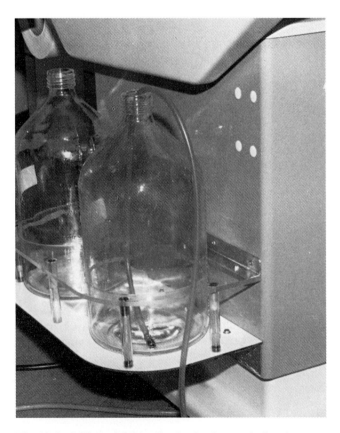

Fig. 11-4. Calibrated fluid collection bottles attached to the gynecologic procedure chair.

COMPLICATIONS FROM IMPAIRED VISUALIZATION

Almost all complications that occur in diagnostic hysteroscopy are caused by improper technique or impaired visualization. Adequate visualization and uterine distention with a clear panoramic view are vitally important for safe hysteroscopic procedures.

To this end the following rules should be kept in mind:

1. Use a good-quality light source, preferably a xenon light with at least 175 W.
2. Check the light cable and telescope if there is a dark image.
3. Always keep the video camera in the upright position; the hysteroscope should be able to rotate freely within the camera coupler. A rotating camera can cause disorientation, resulting in unintentional touching of the endometrium.
4. Do not use CO_2 distention in a bleeding uterus; in this case, use continuous-flow hysteroscopy with pressurized, low-viscosity fluid.
5. In case of impaired visualization caused by blood and/or mucus, flush the uterus with liquid and/or use continuous-flow hysteroscopy.
6. Visualize the endocervical canal and the internal os before inserting the hysteroscope into the uterine cavity.
7. Use the no-touch technique as much as possible.
8. Never advance the hysteroscope with inadequate uterine distention.
9. Never advance the hysteroscope with impaired visualization.

COMPLICATIONS FROM LOCAL ANESTHESIA

In some cases, local anesthesia will be required to reduce patient discomfort, especially when using rigid hysteroscopes in nulliparous and postmenopausal women. We prefer to premedicate all our outpatient hysteroscopy candidates with a prostaglandin synthase inhibitor orally 2 hours before the procedure and 0.5 mg atropine IM 15 minutes before the procedure. This medication prevents painful uterine contractions and vagal reactions during and after the procedure. When local anesthesia is required, the two most important safety precautions are to prevent direct intravascular injection and never exceed the maximum allowed dosage of the agent of choice.

Side effects and toxic reactions

With adequate precautions, side effects and toxic reactions from using local anesthetics will be extremely rare. But when they occur, immediate therapy is vitally important. For this purpose, a complete emergency set should be available in the procedure room.

Toxic reactions can cause either stimulation or depression of the central nervous system. Either effect will occur only with intravascular injection or overdosage. The symptoms can present as acute or late toxic reactions.

The acute toxic reaction includes respiratory arrest, shock, cardiac arrest (CNS depression), or muscular cramps (CNS stimulation). Late toxic reactions generally evoke signs of CNS stimulation such as muscular cramps, reduced vision, nausea, shivering, or convulsions. Sometimes CNS depression such as respiratory or cardiac arrest will also occur.

Therapeutic tools for resuscitation from toxic reactions are a Mayo endotracheal tube, oxygen, and IV access. Medications that should be available include atropine 0.5 mg IV for bradycardia, ephedrine 1 ml IV (50 mg/ml diluted in 9 ml of saline) for hypotension (repeat if necessary), and diazepam (10 to 20 mg IV for severe muscular cramps).

Often the most detrimental side effect of local anesthetics is an allergic reaction, which is very uncommon and requires antiallergic treatment with adrenaline 0.5 ml (1:1000) SQ or IM, clemastine 2 mg IV, prednisolone sodium phosphate 25 mg IV, and supportive measures with IV fluids and oxygen. With bronchospasm, aminophylline 240 mg IV can be administered slowly.

CONCLUSION

Complications during office and outpatient hysteroscopy should be very rare. If they occur, they are almost always caused by lack of experience, improper technique or equipment, or impaired visualization.

By following the rules and precautions for safe hysteroscopic procedures, one can almost always prevent complications. This makes hysteroscopic diagnosis not only a much more reliable but also a much safer procedure than D&C for diagnosing intrauterine disorders in patients with abnormal uterine bleeding and infertility.

REFERENCES

1. Grimes DA: Diagnostic dilatation and curettage: a reappraisal, *Am J Obstet Gynecol* 142:1, 1982.
2. Lindemann HJ: Komplikationen bei der CO_2 Hysteroskopie, *Arch Gynaekol* 219:257, 1975.
3. Lindemann HJ, Mohr J: CO_2 hysteroscopy: diagnosis and treatment, *Am J Obstet Gynecol* 124:129, 1976.
4. Barrôco LE, Oliveira LC, Sá-Melo P: Office hysteroscopy experience with the Hamou microcolpohysteroscope in 250 patients, *Acta Eur Fertil* 17:419, 1986.
5. Raju KS, Taylor RW: Routine hysteroscopy for patients with a high risk of uterine malignancy, *Br J Obstet Gynaecol* 93:1259, 1986.
6. De Jong P, Doel F, Falconer A: Outpatient diagnostic hysteroscopy, *Br J Obstet Gynaecol* 97:299, 1990.
7. Hill NCW et al: Local anaesthesia and cervical dilatation for outpatient diagnostic hysteroscopy, *J Obstet Gynecol* 12:33, 1992.
8. Valle RF: Cervical and uterine complications during insertion of the hysteroscope. In Corfman S, Diamond MP, DeCherney A, Eds: *Complications of laparoscopy and hysteroscopy*, Oxford, 1993, Blackwell Scientific Publications.
9. Wamsteker K, de Blok S: Diagnostic hysteroscopy: technique and documentation. In Sutton C, Diamond MP, Eds: *Endoscopic surgery for gynaecologists*, London, 1993, WB Saunders.
10. Wamsteker K, de Blok S, Emanuel MH: Instrumentation for transcervical hysteroscopic endosurgery, *Gynaecol Endosc* 1:59, 1992.

11. Lindemann HJ et al: Der Einfluss von CO_2 Gas wahrend der Hysteroskopie, *Geburtshilfe Frauenheilkd* 36:153, 1976.

12. Brundin J, Thomassen K: Cardiac gas embolism during carbon dioxide hysteroscopy: risk and management, *Eur J Obstet Gynecol Reprod Biol* 33:241, 1989.

13. Rythen-Alder E et al: Detection of carbon dioxide embolism during hysteroscopy, *Gynaec Endosc* 1:207, 1992.

14. Lukacsko P: Letter, *Fertil Steril* 44:560, 1985.

15. Borton M, Seibert CP, Taymor ML: Recurrent anaphylactic reaction to intraperitoneal dextran 75 used for prevention of postsurgical adhesions, *Obstet Gynecol* 61:755, 1983.

16. Ljungstrom KG et al: Hapten inhibition and dextran anaphylaxis, *Anaesthesia* 43:729, 1988.

Chapter 12

FUTURE OF OFFICE HYSTEROSCOPY

Rafael F. Valle

Although it is easy to look at the past and review the accomplishments and progress that certain techniques and surgical methods have brought to various medical specialties over the years, the future is not always as clear. Nonetheless, the steady and impressive growth of hysteroscopy during the past 25 years can help in predicting the role of office hysteroscopy in the years ahead.

Several large, private consulting firms have estimated that as of 1995 approximately 30% of the 35,000 practicing obstetrician/gynecologists in the United States perform hysteroscopy. Because most diagnostic and therapeutic procedures are performed in the operating room, it has been estimated by a major hysteroscopic manufacturer that only 8% of gynecologists in the United States perform office hysteroscopy. Whether there will be a major migration of procedures to an office-based environment will depend on improved technology, physician education, and reimbursement.

From a technologic perspective, the equipment currently available is more than adequate for office-based diagnostic procedures. As will be discussed later in this chapter, improvements are on the horizon for a variety of hysteroscopes, video systems, and light sources that, when introduced, will allow for a greater number of operative techniques to be performed safely in the office. In general, future generations of hysteroscopes will be smaller, to reduce cervical and uterine pain, will have superior optics, and will allow for continuous fluid flow that will enable office procedures to be performed during minimal to moderate uterine bleeding.

Physician education will be paramount for the movement of hysteroscopy from the operating room to the office. In the future, physicians should be credentialed to perform office hysteroscopy using standards similar to those employed for operative hysteroscopy in the operating room, i.e., attending a didactic/laboratory course, observing several procedures, and having a preceptor observe the first three to five procedures performed in the office by the physician in training. This preceptorship will ensure that the majority of kinks will be eliminated when surgeons learning office hysteroscopy start performing the procedure on their own. Although there is a relatively short learning curve for office hysteroscopy, rigorous training is even more important in the office than in an operating room to minimize the number of complications. The ability to transfer a patient rapidly to an operating room to control a major complication such as bleeding is not always feasible from an office setting.

Ultimately, the greatest influence on the migration of operating room to office-based hysteroscopic procedures may not be what is in the patient's best interest but rather will be physician reimbursement. There is very little doubt that performing hysteroscopic procedures in an office-based environment provides significant savings to the overall health care system. There are substantial savings in anesthesia costs and hospital charges. For example, the total charges for a hospital-based diagnostic hysteroscopy is $2500 to $3000. The total charge for an office hysteroscopy is approximately $450. However, to perform office-based hysteroscopy the health care provider must invest a substantial amount of capital in equipment (see Chapter 3). In the current managed care environment, the migration is reversed. Because they are poorly reimbursed for office-based procedures, physicians have no monetary incentive to perform office hysteroscopy. Because hospitals will pick up the capital equipment costs, physicians have no monetary incentive to invest in these procedures. The office procedures that are being performed are being done because the physicians understand the huge benefits to the patient, i.e., lack of general or regional anesthesia and reduction in postoperative morbidity. However, unless the physician reimbursement system is revised, health care providers may not be able to afford to offer these procedures in the future.

A major driving force to office-based procedures will be capitation. If physicians or hospitals are given a finite amount of money to care for a patient, there is no question the cost savings possible with office-based procedures will become attractive. Capitation will not only influence the growth of office hysteroscopy but also will be the impetus to perform other office-based procedures such as office laparoscopy.

NEED FOR UTERINE EVALUATION

Although the uterus may not seem complex anatomically, no other reproductive organ is as versatile. Because of its varied anatomic, physiologic, and hormonal interactions, the uterus, when afflicted by a pathologic condition, usually manifested by impaired function, abnormal bleeding, and pain, requires meticulous evaluation.[1]

Simple methods of evaluating the uterus involve palpation and visualization of the cervical opening through a vaginal speculum. Advanced methods evaluate uterine size, contours, and volume by abdominal and vaginal sonography and MRI. Before office hysteroscopy, the preferred sequence of evaluation was (1) palpation to assess uterine size, (2) hysterosalpingography to assess the intrauterine cavity, and (3) curettage to assess the endometrial lining.

Palpation to evaluate uterine volume and size can rule out gross changes in the size, contours, and symmetry of the uterine body. However, it may fail to detect smaller lesions within the uterine walls or abnormalities of the uterine cavity, especially the endometrium.

Hysterosalpingography to evaluate the uterine cavity can screen out distortion of symmetry and structural abnormalities. The sensitivity and specificity of this method are reduced by transient uterine cavity distortion, which may be caused by blood clots, mucus, debris, and air bubbles, producing false positive results. Errors in technique, use of radiopaque dye, and interpretation also contribute to failure. Abnormal hysterographic findings have been confirmed by

subsequent hysteroscopy in 43% to 68% of cases in studies comparing these two techniques.[2]

The mechanical curette, introduced by Recamier in 1850,[3] is one of the oldest gynecologic instruments. It is used to sample the endometrium in patients with abnormal uterine bleeding and remove products of conception or pathologic lesions affecting the uterus. Because biopsy of pathologic uterine lesions is unreliable, particularly if the lesions are focal and located at the uterotubal cones, and because structural abnormalities such as leiomyomas and polyps cannot be demonstrated, the value of mechanical curettage has been challenged. Grimes[4] compared the accuracy and adequacy of specimens obtained from mechanical curettage with results obtained by Vabra aspiration. He found more adequate specimens obtained by Vabra aspiration, as well as better accuracy, when compared with specimens obtained with the mechanical curette. As a result of such findings, except when sharp scraping of adherent trophoblastic tissue is required during the removal of products of conception in missed abortion, mechanical curettage has been largely supplanted by aspiration curettage, particularly when done with vacuum suction pumps and flexible plastic cannulas. The trauma of scraping with mechanical curettes, which requires regional or general anesthesia, prompted physicians to use the operating theater for most of these procedures, thereby increasing costs. Finally, the mechanical curette cannot adequately sample the uterine cavity, as demonstrated by studies comparing the accuracy of curettage with subsequent evaluation of the endometrial cavity by hysteroscopy and/or at hysterectomy (Tables 12-1 to 12-3).[5-11]

Table 12-1. Adequacy of dilatation and curettage

Study	Number of patients	Adequate curettage	Incomplete curettage
Englund, S et al,[5] 1957 (D&C/hysteroscopy)	124	44 (35%)	80 (65%)
Gribb, JJ[6] 1960 (D&C/hysteroscopy)	58	9 (15.4%)	49 (84.6%)
Stock, RJ and Kanbour, A,[7] 1975 (D&C/hysterectomy)	50	<½ of cavity in 30 (60%)	⅔ of cavity in 42 (84%)
Word, B et al,[8] 1958 (D&C/hysterectomy)	512	10% of lesions missed by curettage	

Table 12-2. Adequacy of dilatation and curettage for polyps

Study	Number of patients	Diagnosed	Missed
Bibbo, M et al,[9] 1982 (Vakutage/D&C or hysterectomy)	840	83%	17%
Burnett, JE,[10] 1964 (D&C/ hysterectomy)	1298 specimens (121 [9.3%] had polyps)	53%	47%
Grimes, DA,[4] 1982 (Vabra: Review)	111	80%-83%	17%-20%
Valle, RF,[11] 1981 (Hysteroscopy/ D&C)	553 (179 [32.3%] had polyps)	100%/10%	0%/90%

Table 12-3. Adequacy of specimens for endometrial sampling[4]

Dilatation and curettage (2 studies > 300 cases each)	77%-94%
Vabra aspiration (4 studies > 300 cases each)	95%-99%

For many years dilatation and curettage has served as the gold standard for evaluating patients with abnormal uterine bleeding. Although the diagnosis is usually confirmed in this manner, in about 10% of patients the blind curette misses focal pathology, including submucous leiomyomas, endometrial polyps, and occasionally, focal lesions, which may be malignant or premalignant.

In 1935 Novak[12] introduced the metallic aspiration device to avoid cervical dilatation and simplify sampling of the endometrium in patients with abnormal uterine bleeding. New plastic cannulas of small diameter can easily be introduced into the uterine cavity without previous cervical dilatation and, when activated by suction, a satisfactory endometrial sample is obtained. One of the most popular of these devices has been the Vabra device, which has a motor-driven suction unit that produces enough suction to completely denude the entire endometrium for sampling. This method permits easy office sampling of the endometrial lining. Many varieties of devices are based on the same principle and can adequately sample the endometrial cavities of most patients. A new sampling device, the Pipelle, can be used without motorized suction and has been employed in patients without previous cervical dilatation. The suction is induced by a tightly fitted plunger, which is pulled out once the device is in the uterus. This plunger maintains suction while the surgeon, using a rotational motion, withdraws the cannula from the uterine cavity through the cervical canal. One disadvantage of the Pipelle is the poor suction obtained compared with motorized suction units. In addition, because of the cannula's small size, the tissue obtained is much less than what is obtained with plastic cannulas activated by motorized units. A recent controlled study of these devices showed that the Pipelle may provide 10 times less tissue than is obtained by motorized suction devices.[13,14]

Submucous leiomyomas, endometrial polyps, and focal lesions of the endometrium, particularly those contained in polyps or located at the uterotubal cones, may be missed even by these powerful suction devices. It is important to visually inspect the uterine cavity and rule out these abnormal lesions by directed, targeted biopsy of abnormal endometrial areas and/or direct resection of polyps or myomas. MRI is an excellent method of evaluating the uterus because of its precise resolution of the uterine walls and endometrium and its ability to show abnormalities, particularly those that are structural and distort the uterus. MRI is particularly useful in evaluating uterine leiomyomas and adenomyosis, but the expense involved makes it less practical for routine use. It is used only for selected patients.[15]

Because it is noninvasive, sonography (both abdominal and vaginal) affords an excellent evaluation of the uterus, particularly the pregnant uterus. With its high resolution, vaginal sonography can also accurately evaluate the endometrial lining, measuring thickness and distortions by polyps and/or myomas. It is of utmost usefulness in postmenopausal patients, particularly when the endometrial lin-

ing exceeds a thickness of 4 mm as a result of endometrial abnormalities. These patients obviously become excellent candidates for hysteroscopy and selected biopsies.[16] Sonography may not be as useful in the evaluation of premenopausal patients with abnormal uterine bleeding.

ROLE OF DILATATION AND CURETTAGE

Evaluating abnormal uterine bleeding in adult premenopausal and postmenopausal women requires eliminating the possibility of structural abnormalities, as well as abnormal and potentially malignant enodmetrial tissues. Evaluation of the uterus must be simple, effective, and cost efficient. Although the routine use of vaginal sonography accompanied by biopsies may meet the first criterion (simplicity), the abnormal sonographic findings in premenopausal and postmenopausal patients usually require endoscopy to confirm the abnormality and permit targeted biopsies, raising the cost substantially. The use of office hysteroscopy with selected biopsies is simple, is an effective method to rule out structural abnormalities such as myomas, polyps, and focal lesions of the endometrium, and still permits selected targeted biopsies,[17] meeting all three criteria listed above.

At present, the mechanical curette's use as a diagnostic tool has been largely supplanted by suction aspiration devices whose diagnostic accuracy has been enhanced by concomitant visualization of the uterine cavity. The mechanical curette also has been replaced as a therapeutic tool by suction devices, which remove larger portions of the endometrial lining and/or polypoid endometrium than the mechanical curette can. Thus the current roles for the mechanical curette are to dislodge firmly attached trophoblastic tissue from a missed abortion, which is sometimes difficult to remove completely by suction devices, and evacuate thick polypoid endometrium and/or multiple small endometrial polyps. Even in these situations, complete removal of tissue is less than accurate, yielding the view that the mechanical curette is ineffective both for diagnosis and for therapy when compared with newer methods.

Because office hysteroscopy employs small-caliber endoscopes (less than 4 mm O.D.), making cervical dilatation unnecessary generally, examinations are mostly diagnostic. Any pathologic lesions found require either a hysteroscopic biopsy or hysteroscopic removal. Currently, a larger instrument (7 mm O.D.) may be required for operative hysteroscopy performed later in an ambulatory setting under local, regional, or general anesthesia. In the future, improved biopsy instrumentation will allow these lesions to be adequately sampled through a hysteroscope as small as 3.2 mm. Patients with normal findings at hysteroscopy are spared other manipulation or biopsies. At the end of the hysteroscopic examination in a patient with abnormal uterine bleeding and a normal uterine cavity but some irregular desquamation of the endometrial lining on hysteroscopy, a 4-mm soft, plastic cannula is introduced in the uterus, and suction curettage is performed for histologic evaluation of the endometrium (Fig. 12-1).[17-19]

IMPROVEMENTS IN INSTRUMENTATION AND IMAGE CAPABILITIES

Hysteroscopes

Wide-angle optics and excellent resolution can be achieved with today's small (less than 4 mm O.D.) rigid endoscopes. Different adaptors for various light cables can be accommodated. These endoscopes should have a locking mechanism that prevents dislodging the scope's position by inadvertent tripping (Figs. 12-2 to 12-4). Flexible hysteroscopes are also adapted to steer distally but retain rigidity in the main shaft so they can be introduced like the rigid in-

struments. With their 3.6-mm diameter they can be inserted without cervical dilatation. The granular aspect of the image has been refined and is close to the image obtained by rigid endoscopes. These flexible hysteroscopes are totally assembled and come as a single unit.

The next generation of flexible hysteroscopes will have smaller diameters and improved optics. The durometer (stiffness) of the shafts will be somewhere between the very flexible shaft found in the Olympus HYF-P and the rigid shaft in the Fujinon scopes. In addition, the light cord will come as a detachable cable, enabling more convenient cleaning and storage. Other potential improvements include a hysteroscope that is autoclavable and one with an outer sheath that will allow for continuous-flow irrigation of the uterine cavity. Currently available flexible hysteroscopes are

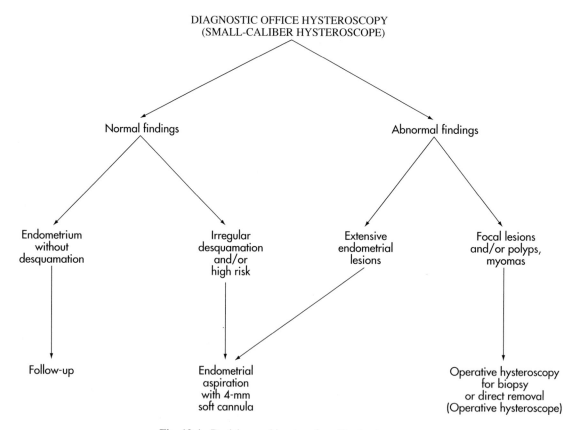

Fig. 12-1. Decision-making tree for office hysteroscopy.

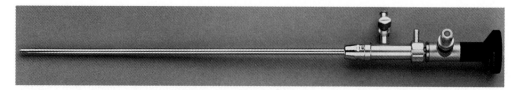

Fig. 12-2. Assembled diagnostic hysteroscope. Telescope with a 2.8 mm O.D. encased in sheath with a 3.3 mm O.D. (Wolf.)

made with valves that must be closed during fluid immersion and opened for gas sterilization. If the valves or caps are in the wrong position, the scopes can sustain significant damage, resulting in expensive repairs. The newer generation of flexible hysteroscopes will have a universal valve that does not need to be adjusted during gas or liquid sterilization.

The contact hysteroscopes introduced in the early 1970s for uterine evaluation did not prove to be practical and accurate tools for systematically evaluating the uterine cavity.[20] The need for contact and segmental evaluation of the uterine lining made contact hysteroscopy less than desirable to evaluate the entire uterus. Borrowing from this method, in 1985 Parent et al,[21] the pioneers of contact hysteroscopy, introduced a new system of uterine evaluation for use in ambulatory patients, specifically in office hysteroscopy. This system, called a *self-contained office hysteroscopy,* incorpo-

rates in a portable unit the endoscope, a cold-light source, and a CO_2 gas insufflator.*

With this isolated system, equipment such as light-transmitting cables, external insufflators, and external light sources can be discarded (Figs. 12-5 to 12-7).

The diagnostic rigid hysteroscope in the self-contained Wolf system has a 3- to 4-mm O.D. The encasing sheath has a 4- to 7-mm O.D. and can be adapted to the telescope and used for diagnosis or therapy. The distention medium flows tangentially along the distal shaft of the telescope, providing a windshield-wiper effect to clear blood and mucus from the endoscope lens. CO_2 is provided by a cartridge or pellet that fits laterally into the insufflator. The pellet contains 4 L of CO_2 under pressure, and the operator regulates the gas pressure and rate of flow. Position 1 delivers gas at 75 cc/minute

*Richard Wolf Medical Instruments Corp., Vernon Hills, Ill., 60061.

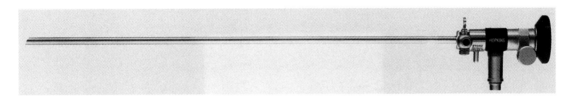

Fig. 12-3. Diagnostic hysteroscope with focusing knob for microhysteroscopy. Telescope with a 4 mm O.D. encased in sheath with a 4.5 mm O.D. (Storz.)

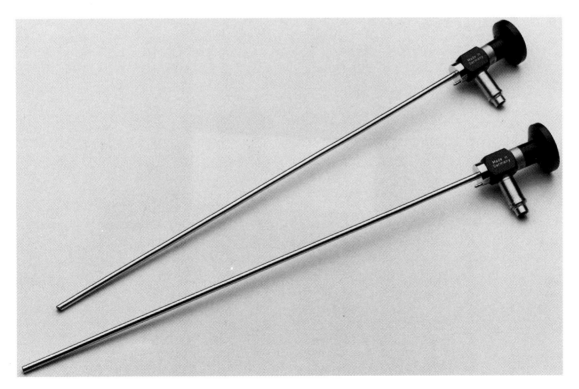

Fig. 12-4. Foreoblique *(top)* and straight view telescopes, 3 mm O.D. for 4 mm O.D. sheaths. (Bryan Corp.)

with an intrauterine pressure of no more than 75 mm Hg. Position 2 delivers the gas at 100 cc/minute with no more than 150 mm Hg pressure. The gas delivery unit has a specially encased self-protection valve to vent the CO_2 in case of failure or excessive pressure.

Light, in this self-contained system, is provided by a miniature projector equipped with a halogen microlamp weighing less than 50 gm. The projector is connected by a cord to the power source, which consists of three rechargeable cadmium-nickel batteries. These batteries are placed in the handle used to direct the instrument. Batteries provide 1 hour of continuous use and are rechargeable.

This hysteroscope is self-contained so manipulation, transport, storage, and care of the instrument are greatly fa-cilitated, making it especially suited for an office setting. The operator must be familiar with the assembly of the instrument and how to adapt flow rates and must check that the batteries are charged before beginning each examination.

Although this self-contained hysteroscopic system is not needed in an office furnished with the necessary equipment to perform conventional office hysteroscopy, it is extremely useful in offices that lack the needed equipment and particularly for physicians who see patients in several office settings. Experience with this type of hysteroscope, especially as a diagnostic tool in the office, has been favorable.

The next generation of rigid office hysteroscopes will have an O.D. of less than 5 mm, provide continuous flow,

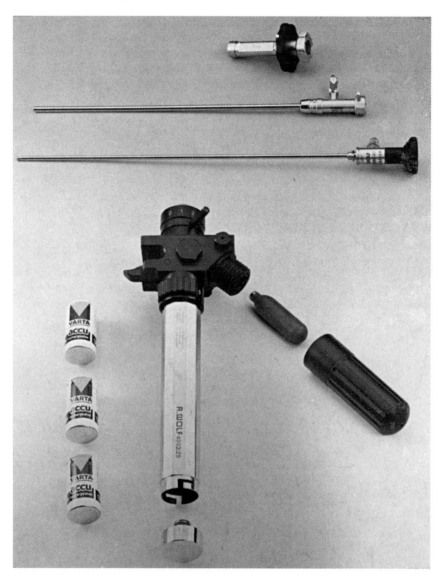

Fig. 12-5. Unassembled, self-contained autonomic hysteroscope. Adaptor, hysteroscopic diagnostic sheath, telescope *(top).* Batteries and gas delivery system *(bottom).* (Wolf.)

and have advanced instrumentation that will allow many operative procedures to be done that now are only performed in the operating room. These newly developed instruments will permit complete and rapid polypectomy, submucous myoma resection or myolysis, and office endometrial ablation. In addition, hysteroscopic GIFT transfers will be safely performed with new catheters specifically developed for these new hysteroscopes.

Video systems

The most significant recent advances in endoscopic technology are the high-resolution cameras of the three-chip or three-dimensional type. These cameras have surpassed natural human ocular resolution and provide magnification that permits identification of small structures and enlargement of the image. These cameras have become indispensable for the endoscopist both for diagnosis and therapeutic procedures (Fig. 12-8).

Video hysteroscopes assembled in one unit will someday facilitate office hysteroscopy by eliminating the need to couple the camera to the endoscope. When the endoscope's ocular apparatus and the still camera are a single unit, the size of the video hysteroscope, the size of the camera, and the weight of the combined unit will decrease. Furthermore, maneuverability will increase, more versatility will be available, and the unit will be simpler to use than those available today.

Digital photography employing laser printers and diskettes has advanced the ability to take serial photographs quickly. It is no longer necessary to stop the procedure and affix the camera to the ocular apparatus of the endoscope. The diskettes permit adequate storage of a large number of pictures, which can later be developed as prints and/or slides for teaching and demonstration (Fig. 12-9).

High-intensity light sources

Intense light sources have been upgraded to provide excellent illumination when using small endoscopes encased in sheaths less than 4 mm in diameter. These light sources, coupled with sensitive video cameras, have provided the best method of practical video hysteroscopy. Water-filled, light-transmitting cables have also added to the intensity of light being provided by these new light sources, complementing the overall system of video hysteroscopy.

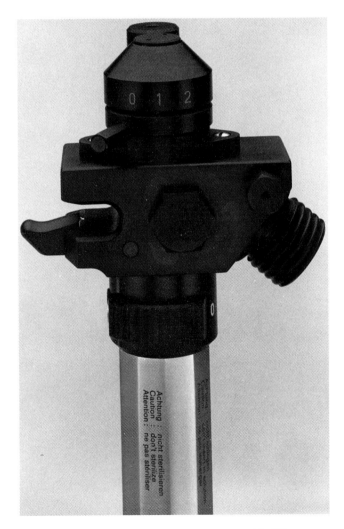

Fig. 12-6. Closer view of gas delivery system with different settings. The battery case acts as a handle. (Wolf.)

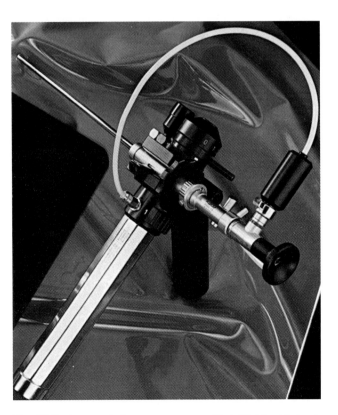

Fig. 12-7. Autonomic hysteroscope assembled. Light cable is attached, and the tubing for CO_2 delivery is connected. (Wolf.)

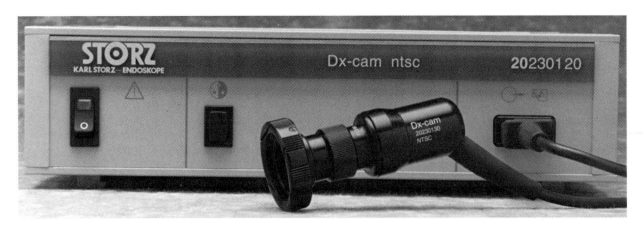

Fig. 12-8. High-sensitivity video camera for office hysteroscopy. (Storz.)

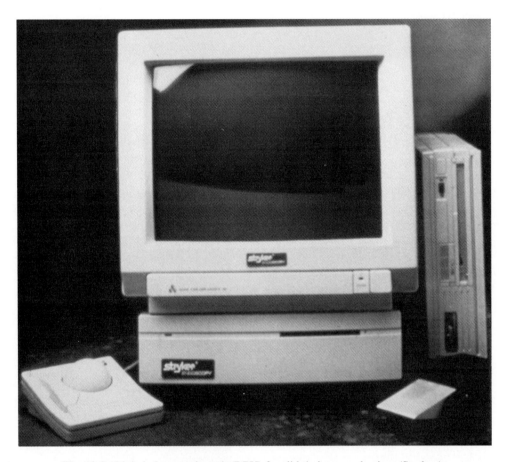

Fig. 12-9. Digital photography unit (DPU) for slide/print reproduction. (Stryker.)

PROCEDURE FOR ROUTINE HYSTEROSCOPY IN EVALUATING ABNORMAL UTERINE BLEEDING

Because of its relative simplicity, safety, and ease, hysteroscopy is applicable as a screening method for patients with abnormal uterine bleeding and/or questionable hysterograms, as well as for patients with suspected intra-

uterine pathology. In the early 1980s small-caliber endoscopes (less than 4 mm O.D.) were introduced for office use that did not require cervical dilatation before being inserted.[22] Their small caliber simplifies their introduction and permits easy and safe investigation of the uterine cavity. Draw-backs to these small-caliber endoscopes include the

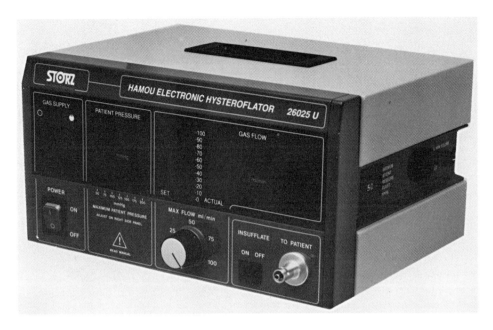

Fig. 12-10. Electronic CO_2 hysteroflator with digital displays of gas flow and intrauterine pressure. (Storz.)

inability to pass instruments through them and to use anything but CO_2 for adequate uterine distention. Their major advantage is that diagnostic hysteroscopy can be performed quickly and simply without the need for anesthesia and analgesia.

The current office hysteroscopes are only appropriate for diagnostic purposes. The distending medium CO_2 is infused with a hysterosufflator (Fig. 12-10), which electronically maintains the flow rate at a constant 40 to 50 cc/minute and permits an intrauterine pressure less than 150 mm Hg, lest the fallopian tubes be open. It should be noted that as the flow rate decreases, the intrauterine pressure increases and vice versa. The patient selected to undergo hysteroscopy requires a pelvic examination and disinfection of the vagina and cervix with an appropriate antiseptic solution such as povidone-iodine. In general, no systemic sedatives or medications are given because the procedure is practically painless. However, a paracervical block using 4 ml of a local anesthetic, such as chloroprocaine hydrochloride (Nesacaine 1%), injected into each uterosacral ligament, and a small dot (0.5 ml) at the site where the tenaculum is to be placed, are useful. Once the anesthetic block is accomplished, a hysteroscope attached to its light source and flowing CO_2 are introduced under direct vision at the ectocervix. The examination begins with slow and systematic filling of the microcavity that the CO_2 produces in front of the endoscope. The endocervical canal is completely explored, then the endoscope is advanced across the internal cervical os. Next the panoramic view of the uterine cavity is evaluated. The uterine cavity is re-examined, as is the endocervical canal, during withdrawal of the instrument.

The original operative hysteroscopes did not provide good inflow and outflow or a continuous-flow system to maintain distention of the uterine cavity and permit continuous irrigation and washing of the cavity. Today hysteroscopy can be performed in an office using a continuous-flow operative hysteroscope with an O.D. of up to 5.5 mm, but the cervical dilatation and manipulation needed for this size instrument require added personnel and attention to detail, as well as safety measures in anticipation of side effects such as bradycardia and hypotension. The procedure is similar to the one just detailed, but the endocervical canal is gradually dilated to number 6 Hegar or to the exact diameter of the specific operative hysteroscope being used. A cervical cap is not required; it is cumbersome to apply and cannot prevent reflux of the distending medium, including gas. Despite the feasibility of introducing an operative hysteroscope under the paracervical local anesthesia, most operative procedures performed in the office are limited to removal of IUDs, biopsy of focal lesions, removal of some polyps, and tubal occlusion procedures, along with a few others. Unless performed by experienced hysteroscopists (see Chapter 10), extended manipulation and surgical interventions, such as division of extensive uterine adhesions, division of uterine septa, or removal of submucous leiomyomas, are more safely and effectively done while the patient is under general anesthesia and, in some instances, with concomitant laparoscopy.

Hysteroscope suction aspiration sampling may be used to evaluate patients with abnormal uterine bleeding in whom no specific lesions were discovered by visualization and no targeted selected biopsies or treatment of specific lesions is required. This technique offers accurate evaluation of the

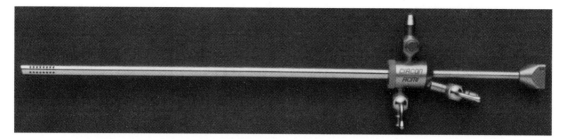

Fig. 12-11. Continuous-flow diagnostic sheath, 5.5 mm O.D. with an operating channel 1 mm in diameter. (Circon Corp.)

uterine cavity for structural abnormalities such as endometrial polyps, submucous leiomyomas, and/or focal lesions of the endometrium; furthermore, it provides an excellent sampling of endometrial tissue. When targeted biopsies or selected treatment is required, the diagnostic hysteroscope (which is less than 4 mm O.D.) will be replaced by the operative hysteroscope, and cervical dilatation will be necessary.

In summary, office hysteroscopy is a simple procedure that can be undertaken in a short time with minimal morbidity and inconvenience to the patient. The patient must be selected carefully and the examination strictly timed to the early follicular phase once menstruation has ceased. When suction, motor-driven, plastic cannulas are added for endometrial sampling and in the absence of focal lesions, hysteroscopy with a small (less than 4 mm O.D.) instrument is an excellent method for evaluating abnormal uterine bleeding that is unresponsive to hormonal therapy.

OPERATIVE PROCEDURES THAT MAY SOON BE PERFORMED IN THE OFFICE

New instrumentation, such as outflow sheaths, allow continuous-flow washing of the uterine cavity without exceeding the 5.5-mm O.D. of the hysteroscope, permitting a faster, safer, and more effective method of performing minor operations in the office (Figs. 12-11 and 12-12). These procedures include removal of small endometrial polyps and submucous leiomyomas of the pedunculated type, division of focal intrauterine adhesions, selective biopsies of abnormal areas, and removal of misplaced or "lost" foreign bodies such as IUDs. When technology provides a simple, effective, and safe method of tubal occlusion, tubal sterilization may also be performed in the office.

To make office hysteroscopy still more versatile, particularly for therapeutic uses, instrumentation must be further modified and enhanced. Micromorcellators, driven hydraulically or electronically, will need to be adapted to hysteroscopes of less than 6 mm O.D. to avoid excessive cervical dilatation and facilitate the treatment of some minor conditions. Limited manipulation will be needed so that the operation can be performed safely and effectively.

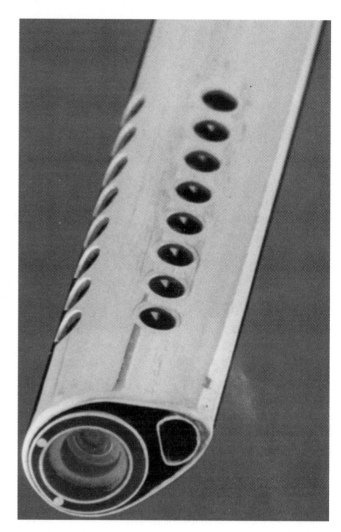

Fig. 12-12. Close-up view of continuous-flow diagnostic sheath with telescope in place. Inflow adjacent to telescope, outflow from distal fenestrations on sheath. (Circon Corp.)

To expand the therapeutic uses of office hysteroscopic procedures, patient selection, procedure, and instrumentation should be rigidly controlled by the practitioner, whose criteria should be to select simple, easy, and nonrisky cases that can indeed be performed in the office better than in the

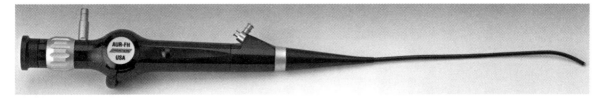

Fig. 12-13. Flexible diagnostic hysteroscope (AUR-FH), 2.8 mm O.D. (Circon Corp.)

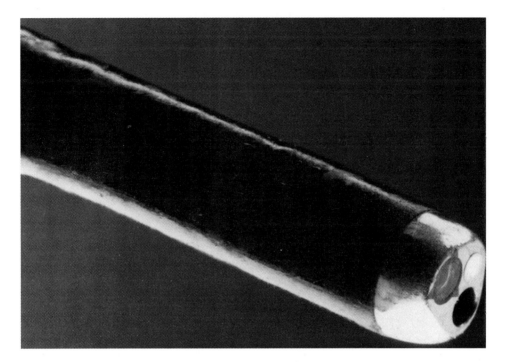

Fig. 12-14. Close-up view of distal end of flexible hysteroscope. (Circon Corp.)

operating theater. Office operative hysteroscopy should not be viewed as a way to impress patients and peers or test the ability to bypass common sense and clinical judgment. Realistically, hysteroscopic procedures that could become office-based may involve two approaches to the fallopian tube: tubal cannulation to implement new reproductive technologies, such as GIFT, ZIFT and direct tubal insemination[23]; and tubal sterilization, should a practical, simple, and effective hysteroscopic method ever be developed to effect not only permanent but also even temporary tubal sterilization that can be reversed without damage (box and Figs. 12-13 and 12-14).[24] In addition, office falloposcopy may find real value in the routine evaluation of infertile patients with tubal factor or unexplained infertility (see Chapter 13).

The introduction of small resectoscopes (less than 6 mm O.D.) with continuous-flow systems and electrodes shaped variously to adapt to the operation being performed will also enhance the applications of office hysteroscopic procedures.

Future applications of office hysteroscopy

Study of endometrial surface changes in various phases of the menstrual cycle

Study of intratubal milieu, biochemistry of tubal secretions, and tubal motility with open-ended catheters

Delivery of flexible miniendoscopes at the uterotubal junctions for intratubal observations

Tubal occlusion by electrocoagulation, cryocoagulation, instillation of chemical substances, or placement of mechanical plugs

Application of new reproductive technologies (intratubal insemination, GIFT, ZIFT)

Study of endometrium to assess adequate maturity prior to IVF-ET

Chorionic villus sampling under hysteroscopy

Embryoscopy-fetoscopy

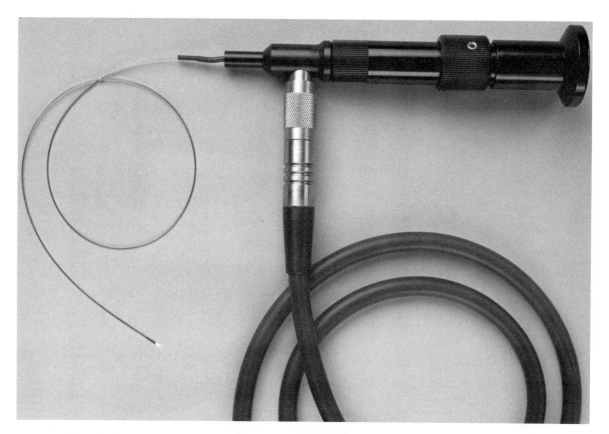

Fig. 12-15. Assembled falloposcope, 0.5 mm diameter, with ocular portion and light-transmitting cable. (Ova Medical Corp.)

Lasers, particularly fiber-lasers, remain promising as a source of energy for therapeutic uses, particularly because of the relative ease in manipulating the fibers through small endoscopes. However, major modifications and advances in present technology must occur to make them portable, easy to store, less complex to maintain, and perhaps even tuneable. The expense involved in acquiring these units must markedly decrease to make them practical, affordable, and cost effective. Free-electron lasers and dye lasers could revolutionize the current therapeutic approach to the uterus. As discussed by in Chapter 14, selective local sensitization of tissues with hematoporphyrin derivatives (HPD) could also expand the applications of dye lasers for office endometrial ablation.[25]

As miniaturization of instruments evolves further, transcervical embryoscopy and selective chorionic villus sampling may become realities.[26,27] Fiberoptic miniendoscopes (less than 0.5 mm in diameter) with enhanced resolution may eventually provide acceptable images to accurately evaluate the fallopian tubes transcervically. They would be usable through small hysteroscopes and would not require cervical dilatation for introduction, making salpingoscopy practical and reproducible in the office (Figs. 12-15 and 12-16).

CONCLUSION

Office hysteroscopy is a simple procedure that can be undertaken in a short time with minimal morbidity and inconvenience to the patient. It is important to perform an examination in the early follicular phase once menstruation has ceased. When plastic cannulas are used as an adjunct to hysteroscopy for endometrial sampling, the procedure offers an excellent method to evaluate patients with abnormal uterine bleeding that is unresponsive to hormonal therapy. The use of hysteroscopy with selected biopsies for the evaluation of patients with abnormal uterine bleeding has added to the accuracy and completeness of this evaluation to rule out structural abnormalities and abnormal endometrial focal lesions that can be missed by blind methods of evaluation.

Because of better instrumentation and continuous-flow hysteroscopes, therapeutic procedures such as tubal cannulation for implementation of new reproductive technologies such as GIFT and ZIFT may easily be performed in an office. Eventually, tubal sterilization may also be performed as an office procedure if a safe and effective method is found. Office hysteroscopy should be adopted by every gynecologist as an excellent method of routine uterine evaluation.

New technology may provide a way to perform minor therapeutic procedures, such as removal of small polyps and

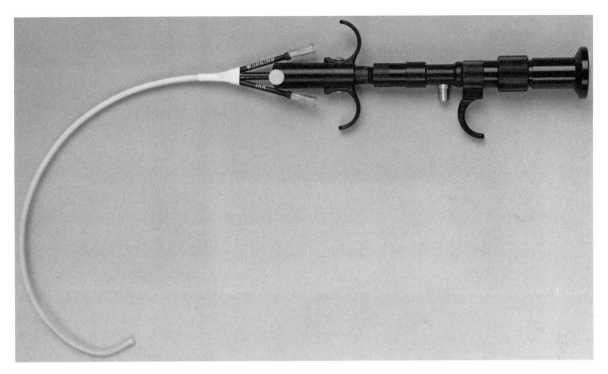

Fig. 12-16. Flexible hysteroscope, 1 mm diameter, in a 3.7-mm O.D. disposable sheath with a 1-mm inner diameter channel for instrumentation and a 1.3-mm inner diameter channel for telescope and irrigation. (Ova Medical Corp.)

submucous leiomyomas, division of focal intrauterine adhesions, and treatment of small uterine septa, in the office in a safe, effective, and practical manner. Still on the horizon are falloposcopy, transcervical embryoscopy, and chorionic villus sampling.

The future of office hysteroscopy is bright and promising, particularly in defining its rightful place in evaluating patients with abnormal uterine bleeding.

REFERENCES

1. Valle RF: Clinical management of uterine factors in infertile patients. In Speroff, L, Ed: *Seminars in Reproductive Endocrinology,* New York, 1985, Thieme-Stratton, Inc., George Thieme Verlag.
2. Valle RF, Sciarra JJ: Current status of hysteroscopy in gynecologic practice, *Fertil Steril* 32:619, 1979.
3. Leonardo RA: *History of gynecology.* New York, 1944, Froben Press.
4. Grimes DA: Diagnostic dilatation and curettage: a reappraisal, *Am J Obstet Gynecol* 142:1, 1982.
5. Englund SE et al: Hysteroscopy in diagnosis and treatment of uterine bleeding, *Gynecologia* 143:217, 1957.
6. Gribb JJ: Hysteroscopy: an aid in gynecologic diagnosis, *Obstet Gynecol* 15:593, 1960.
7. Stock RJ, Kanbour A: Prehysterectomy curettage, *Obstet Gynecol* 45:537, 1975.
8. Word B, Gravlee LC, Wideman GL: The fallacy of simple uterine curettage, *Obstet Gynecol* 12:642, 1958.
9. Bibbo M et al: Accuracy of three sampling techniques for the diagnosis of endometrial cancer and hyperplasias, *J Reprod Med* 27:622, 1982.
10. Burnett JE: Hysteroscopy-controlled curettage for endometrial polyps, *Obstet Gynecol* 24:621, 1964.
11. Valle RF: Hysteroscopic evaluation of patients with abnormal uterine bleeding, *Surg Gynecol Obstet* 153:521, 1981.
12. Novak E: A suction-curet apparatus for endometrial biopsy, *JAMA* 104:1794, 1935.
13. Rodriguez GC, Yakub N, King ME: A comparison of the Pipelle device and the Vabra aspiration as measured by endometrial denudation in hysterectomy specimens: the Pipelle device samples significantly less of the endometrial surface than the Vabra aspirator, *Am J Obstet Gynecol* 168:55, 1993.
14. Goldchmit R et al: The accuracy of endometrial Pipelle sampling with and without sonographic measurement of endometrial thickness, *Obstet Gynecol* 82:727, 1993.
15. Binkovitz LA, King BF: Advances in gynecologic imaging and intervention, *Mayo Clin Proc* 16:1133, 1991.
16. Goldstein SR et al: Endometrial assessment of vaginal ultrasonography before endometrial sampling in patients with postmenopausal bleeding, *Am J Obstet Gynecol* 163:119, 1990.
17. Valle RF: Hysteroscopy. In Garcia CR, Mastroianni L, Amelar RD, and Dubin L, Eds: *Current therapy of infertility,* Toronto, Philadelphia, 1988, B.C. Decker, Inc.
18. Font-Sastre V et al: Office hysteroscopy with small calibre instruments, *Acta Eur Fertil* 17:413, 1986.
19. Goldrath MH, Sherman AI: Office hysteroscopy and suction curettage: can we eliminate the hospital diagnostic D&C?, *Am J Obstet Gynecol* 152:220, 1985.
20. Barbot J: Contact hysteroscopy: Another method of endoscopic examination of the uterine cavity, *Am J Obstet Gynecol* 136:721, 1980.
21. Parent B et al: In Meloine, SA, Ed: *Panoramic hysteroscopy,* Paris, 1985, English translated edition distributed by Williams and Wilkins, Baltimore, 1987.
22. Hamou J: Microhysteroscopy: a new procedure and its original applications in gynecology, *J Reprod Med* 26:375, 1981.
23. Valle RF: Future growth and development of hysteroscopy, *Obstet Gynecol Clin North Am* 15:107-126, 1988.

24. Valle RF: Hysteroscopic sterilization. In Baggish MS, Barbot J, and Valle RF, Eds: *Diagnostic and operative hysteroscopy,* St. Louis, 1989, Mosby-Year Book.

25. Battha N et al: Endometrial ablation by means of photodynamic therapy with photofrin II, *Am J Obstet Gynecol* 167:1856, 1992.

26. Nordenskjold F, Gustavii B: Direct-vision chorionic villi biopsy for prenatal diagnosis in first trimester, *J Reprod Med* 29:572, 1984.

27. Gustavii B: Direct vision technique for chorionic villi sampling in 100 diagnostic cases. In Fraccaro M et al, Eds: *First trimester fetal diagnosis,* Berlin, 1985, Springer-Verlag.

Chapter 13

OFFICE FALLOPOSCOPY

Eric S. Surrey

Falloposcopy is a transcervical, transvaginal approach for visualizing the fallopian tubal lumen from the uterotubal junction to the fimbria. The first reports of the successful use of this microendoscopic technique were provided in 1990 by Kerin et al.[1,2] Although the majority of the data regarding both diagnostic and therapeutic applications of falloposcopy were derived from procedures performed under general anesthesia in a hospital, the potential for office-based falloposcopy is great.

INDICATIONS AND CONTRAINDICATIONS FOR OFFICE FALLOPOSCOPY

The primary indication for performing outpatient falloposcopy, as shown in the box on page 132, is to assess the infertile woman with suspected proximal tubal disease after a hysterosalpingogram or in whom hysterosalpingography is contraindicated. The poor correlation between findings at hysterosalpingography and surgery, particularly with regard to proximal tubal occlusion, has been reported by Sulak et al.[3] Before subjecting a patient to microsurgical anastomosis at laparotomy or tubal bypass employing the assisted reproductive technologies, a thorough assessment of the tubal lumen may reveal findings such as spasm of the uterotubal ostium (UTO), intralumenal polyps, or mucous plugs, which may lend themselves to less invasive therapy. Similarly, the finding of an irreparably damaged tubal lumen may allow the patient to avoid laparoscopy altogether and be referred directly for IVF-ET.

The patient with hydrosalpinges diagnosed radiologically may also benefit from this outpatient procedure. Although falloposcopy provides no information regarding peritubal disease, should the endothelial lining prove to be damaged beyond repair, further surgical investigation would be unwarranted. In contrast, a patient with less severely damaged endothelial lining noted at falloposcopy could then be scheduled for a laparoscopic procedure to assess the extent of peritubal disease and potentially perform endoscopic tubal reconstruction.

A third indication is the patient with otherwise unexplained infertility after a standard evaluation. Patients with normal findings at hysterosalpingography and laparoscopy have been noted to have intralumenal adhesions and abnormal endothelial vascular patterns during tubal microendoscopy.[4] In addition, the use of falloposcopic visualization of the tubal lumen to confirm appropriate catheter placement before outpatient transcervical gamete transfer has been reported.[5]

Contraindications to office-based falloposcopy are also displayed in the box. This procedure should not be performed in the face of active pelvic infection or uterine bleeding, or in patients unable to tolerate local anesthetic agents. Patients with endometrial pathology such as synechiae or submucous myoma preventing visualization and access to the uterotubal ostium are poor candidates as well.

TECHNIQUE

Patient preparation

Falloposcopy is most easily performed during the mid-follicular phase of the menstrual cycle after cessation of menses. Patients are given antibiotics prophylactically. In their series on outpatient falloposcopy, Scudamore, Dunphy, and Cooke[6] administered naproxen, diazepam, and uterosacral lidocaine as anesthesia to 14 patients after dissatisfaction with 2 other regimes in 7 other patients. In contrast, Venezia et al[7] premedicated eight patients examined in an outpatient setting with atropine sulfate and benzodiazepine without complication. Dunphy[8] employed intravenous fentanyl and benzodiazepine with similar success. Intraoperative monitoring of patients with pulse oximetry, combined with frequent recordings of

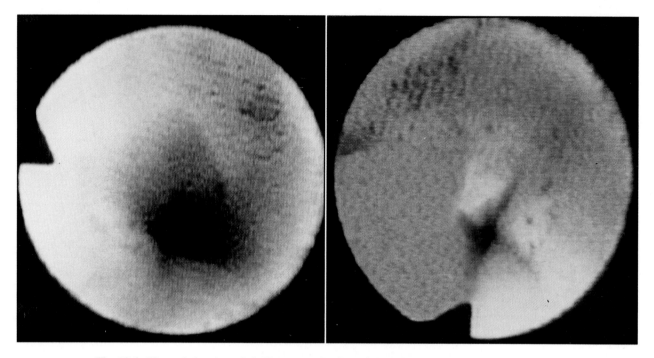

Fig. 13-1. Uterotubal ostium. *Left,* Hysteroscopic view of the UTO in a relaxed state. *Right,* Hysteroscopic view of the same UTO 2 seconds later while contracting. Note the pucker appearance. (Reprinted with permission from Kerin JF et al: *Fertil Steril* 54:390-400, 1990, Fig. 4.)

Indications for office falloposcopy

1. Suspected proximal tubal occlusion
2. Suspected distal tubal occlusion
3. Unexplained infertility
4. Contraindication to hysterosalpingography (contrast dye allergy)
5. Gamete and/or zygote transfer?

Contraindications to office falloposcopy

1. Active pelvic infection
2. Active uterine bleeding
3. Allergic reaction to local anesthetic agents
4. Extensive uterine synechiae or submucous myomata

blood pressure and pulse, provide additional safety. Patients should have their vital signs monitored and be allowed to recover for 1 hour after the procedure.

Coaxial technique

With use of the coaxial method[1,2] for performing falloposcopy, the uterotubal ostium is first visualized by introducing a flexible hysteroscope into the endometrial cavity under video monitoring to achieve a long-axis view within 1 to 2 mm of the tubal ostia. Cervical dilation is rarely required and should be avoided if possible to prevent leakage. A variety of hysteroscopes with O.D.s of 1.5 to 2 mm and a single operating channel have been employed.* Lactated Ringer's

solution is infused as a distention medium through extension tubing connected to one arm of an attached Tuohy-Borst Y-connector.† A flexible, platinum-tipped, tapered guidewire of 0.3 to 0.8 mm O.D‡ is then introduced into the UTO through the second arm of the Y-connector and advanced until either a point of resistance, increase in patient discomfort, or a distance of 15 cm is reached. Care should be taken to avoid passage of the wire through the UTO during a period of ostial spasm (Fig. 13-1). It should be noted that although the intramural segment of the fallopian tube is fairly straight over its 1.5- to 2.5-cm length, it may form an acute angle with the cavity. A gentle torque motion may facilitate guidewire passage through this region.

Once the wire has been introduced, a Teflon-coated catheter with a 1.2- to 1.3-mm O.D.§ is introduced over the wire for a similar distance (Fig. 13-2). The guidewire is then withdrawn.

A second Tuohy-Borst Y-connector is then attached to the proximal end of the catheter. The falloposcope is introduced through the straight arm of the second Y-connector. This allows protection for the atraumatic leading end of the highly flexible falloposcope, which measures 120 to 130 cm in length, and 0.3 to 0.5 mm in O.D.i The coaxial system is dis-

*Olympus Corp., Lake Success, N.Y.; Intramed Laboratories, San Diego, Calif.; Mitsubishi Cable Industries, Itami, Japan.

†Cook OB-GYN, Spencer, Ind.
‡Target Therapeutics, San Jose, Calif.; Conceptus, Inc., San Carlos, Calif.; Cook OB-GYN, Spencer, Ind.; Glidewire Medi-Tech, Watertown, N.H.
§Target Therapeutics, San Jose, Calif.; Conceptus, Inc., San Carlos, Calif.; Cook OB-GYN, Spencer, Ind.
iOlympus Corp., Lake Success, N.Y.; Mitsubishi Cable Industries, Itami, Japan; Intramed Laboratories, San Diego, Calif.; Medical Dynamics, Inc., Englewood, Colo.

played in Fig. 13-3. Lactated Ringer's solution is infused through the angled arm of this second Y-connector. A xenon light source, camera chip, and high-resolution video monitor are required. Visualization of the tubal lumen is performed in a retrograde fashion, taking care to maintain the falloposcope flush with the distal opening of the catheter. A white-out will occur if the lens directly touches the tubal endothelial lining. Dual video monitoring of hysteroscopy and falloposcopy is helpful. This technique is summarized in the box on page 134. The use of this technique in an office setting requires the infusion of minimal amounts of distending medium and extremely gentle incremental movement of catheters and guidewires.

Linear everting catheter system technique

The linear everting catheter (LEC) system* represents an alternative approach for transcervical cannulation and visualization of the fallopian tubal lumen.[9] The majority of experience with office falloposcopy has been achieved with this device.[6-11] The LEC consists of an outer and inner catheter body that is joined distally by a balloon (Fig. 13-4). This balloon everts by pressurization of a joining membrane, which slowly unrolls the catheter tip as the inner body is advanced.

*Imagyn, Laguna Niguel, Calif.

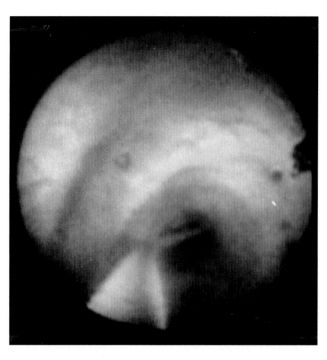

Fig. 13-2. Catheterization of the UTO with instillation of dilute indigo carmine dye during selective chromotubation before falloposcopy. (Courtesy John Kerin, M.D., Ph.D.)

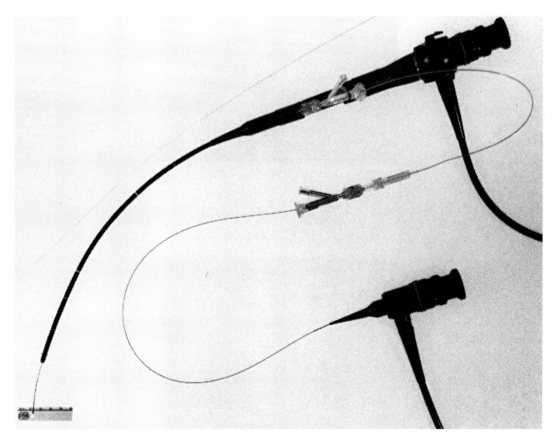

Fig. 13-3. Coaxial falloposcopy. Falloposcope has been placed through straight arm of Y-connector into Teflon over-the-wire catheter. The catheter has been previously introduced through the operating channel of the flexible hysteroscope.

The UTO is visualized by introducing the falloposcope through the distal lumen of the catheter, thus obviating the need for a separate hysteroscope. The balloon is pressurized and the catheter slowly everted. This catheter system allows the balloon to more accurately conform to the tortuous path of the fallopian tube while eliminating lateral shear forces. When the tube has been *completely* catheterized to the point at which resistance is met or when the catheter has been advanced 15 cm, the 0.5-mm O.D. falloposcope is subsequently introduced through the everted catheter. Falloposcopy is also performed in a retrograde fashion. Discomfort can be minimized by slow, incremental eversion of the catheter. Patient acceptance can also be enhanced by use of minimal amounts of flush in a slow, continuous fashion during retrograde falloposcopy.

Normal anatomy

The endothelial lining of the intramural portion of the fallopian tube ranges from 0.8 to 1 mm in diameter and is marked by several flattened folds. The isthmic region extends for 2 to 3 cm, with a diameter of 1 to 2 mm, and is marked by 4 to 6 longitudinal folds with a more delicate vascular pattern (Fig. 13-5). The ampulla rapidly increases in diameter from 1.5 to 4 mm proximally to 8 to 10 mm distally. Its variable length ranges from 5 to 10 cm. Progressing distally, one can visualize a radial pattern of primary folds 4 mm in height that increase in number (Fig. 13-6). As one reaches the more distal aspects of the ampullary region, one can discern delicate secondary folds that have a fine vascular pattern.

Pathologic findings

A variety of pathologic findings within the tubal lumen have been effectively visualized with the aid of transcervical falloposcopy. Distally, one is able to assess the extent of inflammatory vascular patterns, mucosal atrophy, and loss of primary endothelial folds characteristic of hydrosalpinges (Fig. 13-7). More proximal lesions that can be seen include varying degrees of stenoses, nonocclusive intralumenal adhesions, tubal polyps, mucous plugs, and the endothelial diverticulae associated with salpingitis isthmica nodosa (Figs. 13-8 to 13-10).

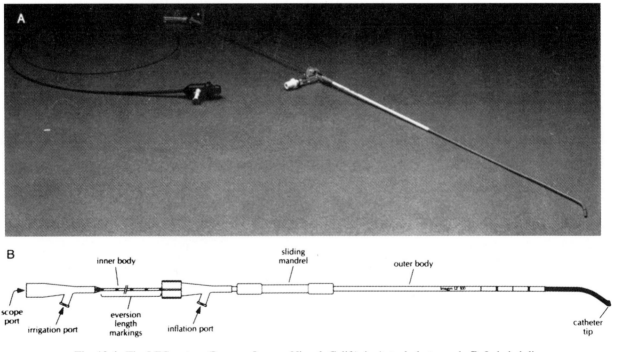

Fig. 13-4. The LEC system (Imagyn, Laguna Niguel, Calif.) **A,** Actual photograph. **B,** Labeled diagram. (Reprinted with permission from Pearlstone AC et al: *Fertil Steril* 58:854-7, 1992, Fig. 1.)

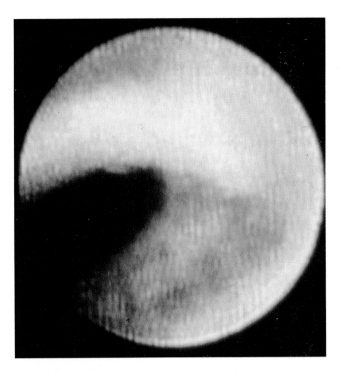

Fig. 13-5. Falloposcopic image of the normal tubal isthmus obtained with the LEC. (Reprinted with permission from Pearlstone AC et al: *Fertil Steril* 58:854-7, 1992, Fig. 3A.)

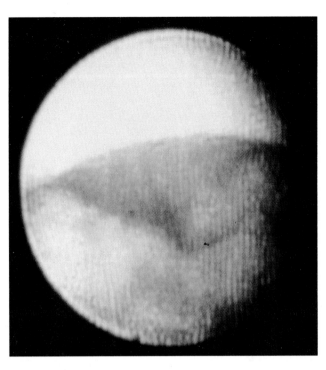

Fig. 13-6. Falloposcopic image of the normal tubal ampulla obtained with the LEC. (Reprinted with permission from Pearlstone AC et al: *Fertil Steril* 58:854-7, 1992, Fig. 3B.)

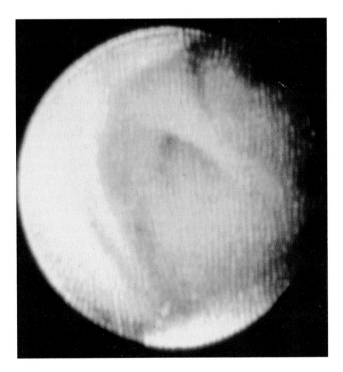

Fig. 13-7. Hydrosalpinx visualized with the LEC. Note flattened fibrotic endothelial lining. (Reprinted with permission from Pearlstone et al: *Fertil Steril* 58:854-7, 1992, Fig. 3C.)

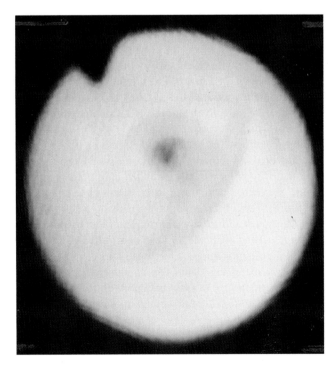

Fig. 13-8. Isthmic stenosis visualized with coaxial falloposcopy system.

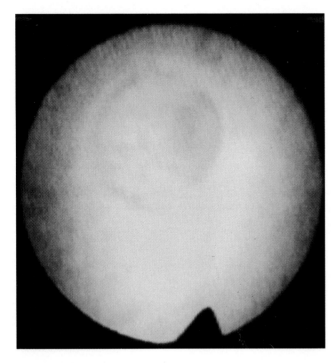

Fig. 13-9. Complete isthmic obstruction visualized with coaxial falloposcopy system.

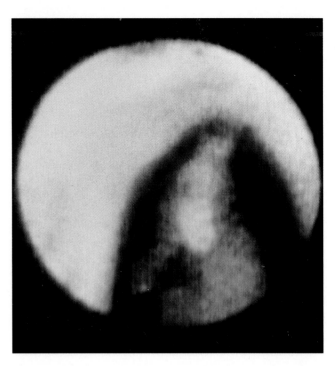

Fig. 13-10. Endothelial polyp causing partial tubal obstruction visualized with coaxial falloposcopy system. (Reprinted with permission from Kerin J et al: *Fertil Steril* 57:731-41, 1992, Fig. 5.)

Kerin et al[12] have devised a classification and scoring system to both standardize and validate these findings (Fig. 13-11). This scoring system attributes points to each segment of the fallopian tube for patency, intralumenal adhesions, extent of dilation, and quality of the ruggal folds and vascular patterns. In a recent series describing the results of falloposcopic assessment of 112 tubes in 75 women with a provisional radiologic diagnosis of tubal disease, severe obstructive disease was noted in 25% of the tubes, mild to moderate disease in 29%, and no disease in 46%.[12] Grow, Coddington, and Flood[13] performed falloposcopy in 12 tubes noted to be proximally occluded at hysterosalpingography. Nine tubes were noted to be patent at falloposcopy. Only three were observed to have a discrete obstructive lesion. Venezia et al[7] recently reported that falloposcopic findings appreciated with the LEC system failed to correlate with hysterosalpingographic findings in 40% of tubes visualized. It is interesting to note that in our series, pregnancies were achieved in 21% of those patients with at least one normal tube, in 9% (2/72) of those with moderate disease, and in none of the 16 patients with severe disease. Larger scale trials with longer term follow-up are under way to substantiate the predictive validity of this system.

Complications

Office-based falloposcopy has only been described with use of the LEC system in published series to date.[6-11] Scudamore, Dunphy, and Cooke[6] were able to successfully perform bilateral tubal endoscopic visualization in 18 of 19

patients with a mean operating time of 35 minutes (range was 25 to 50 minutes). Of 37 tubes visualized, 34 showed epithelial characteristics. No complications were reported. Bauer et al[10] performed outpatient falloposcopy in 8 tubes in 7 patients before intratubal insemination. No irrigation was employed within the tube, and falloposcopy was performed solely to confirm catheter location within the tube. Catheterization was successfully performed in all patients without complications. Dunphy[8] reported that in-office falloposcopy induced significantly less intense pain than hysterosalpingography. Rapid eversion, cannulation, and flushing near the UTO were associated with the most severe discomfort in this series. In an additional report, Dunphy et al[11] described successful outpatient LEC falloposcopy in 24 of 25 fallopian tubes without complication. The mean duration of the procedures was 29 minutes. In our experience with the LEC performing falloposcopy under general anesthesia, 95.6% (43/45) of tubes in 26 women were successfully cannulated.[9] Adequate imaging was achieved in 90.6% (39/43). Employing a coaxial technique, we recently reported an inability to advance the falloposcope or visualize the fallopian tubal lumen in the absence of detectable lesions in only 10/131 (8.5%) of tubes.[14]

The primary risk of falloposcopy is tubal perforation, although its incidence is extremely low.[15] The most common sites for tubal perforation are displayed in Fig. 13-12. Exaggerated acute angles formed by the junction of the intramural portion of the tube with the UTO, peritubal adhesions limiting tubal flexibility, and narrowing of the lumen be-

FALLOPOSCOPIC CLASSIFICATION, SCORING AND LOCALIZATION OF TUBAL LUMEN DISEASE

Patient's Name _____ Date _____ Phone # _____
Age _____ G _____ P _____ SAB _____ TAB _____ Ectopic _____ Infertile: Yes _____ No _____
Other Significant History (i.e. surgery, infection, etc.) _____
_____

HSG _____ Sonography _____ Photography _____ Laparoscopy _____ Laparotomy _____
Cycle Details _____
Saman Details _____

SITE of DISEASE	RIGHT TUBE				LEFT TUBE			
	INTRAMURAL	ISTHMIC	AMPULLARY	FIMBRIAL	INTRAMURAL	ISTHMIC	AMPULLARY	FIMBRIAL
PATENCY Patency __ __ __ __ 1 Stenosis __ __ __ __ 2 Fibrotic obstruction __ __ 3								
EPITHELIUM Normal __ __ __ __ 1 Pale, Atropic __ __ __ 2 Flat, featureless __ __ 3								
VASCULARITY Normal __ __ __ __ 1 Intermediate __ __ __ 2 Poor pallor __ __ __ 3								
ADHESIONS None __ __ __ __ 1 Thin, weblike __ __ __ 2 Thick __ __ __ __ 3								
DILITATION None __ __ __ __ 1 Minimal __ __ __ __ 2 Hydrosalpinx __ __ __ 3								
*OTHER __ __ __ 2–3								
CUMULATIVE SCORE								

TOTAL SCORE   RIGHT TUBE = _____   (NORMAL = 20)   LEFT TUBE = _____   (NORMAL = 20)

A cumulative score for each tube of: 20 = Normal Tubal Lumen; >20 but <30 = Moderate Endotubal Disease; >30 = Severe Endotubal Disease.
* Mucus Plugs or Tubal Debris, Endotubal Polyps, Endometriosis, Salpingitis Isthmica Nodosa, Inflammatory, Infectious, Neoplastic
  conditions and absent tubal segments are each assigned a score of 2 to 3 depending on the significance of the lesion.

Treatment (Specify R & L Tube Surgical Procedures).

Nothing _____
Aquadissection _____
Guidewire Cannulation _____
Wire Dilitation _____
Direct Balloon Tuboplasty _____
Other _____

Prognosis for Conception:

_____ Excellent (>75%)
_____ Good (50–75%)
_____ Fair (25–50%)
_____ Poor (<25%)

Recommended Followup Treatment: _____
_____
_____

Surgeons _____
_____
_____
_____

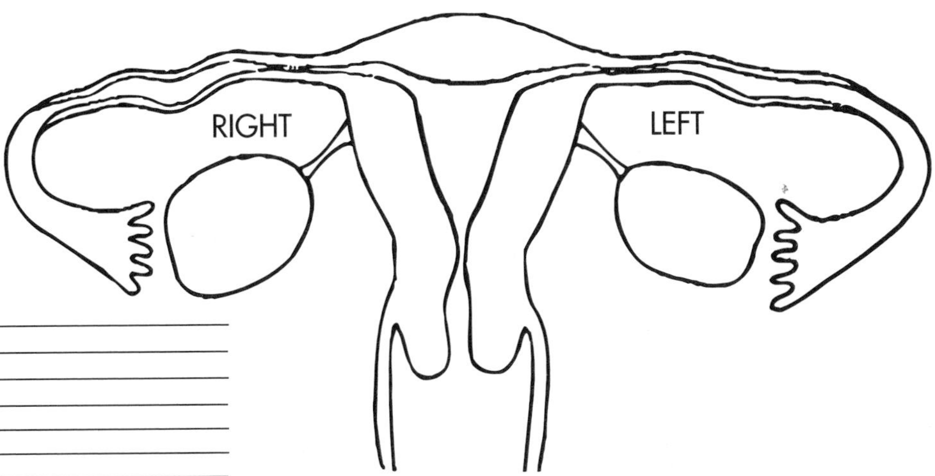

Fig. 13-11. Classification system for falloposcopic findings. (Reprinted with permission from Kerin J et al: *Fertil Steril* 57:731-41, 1992, Fig. 1.)

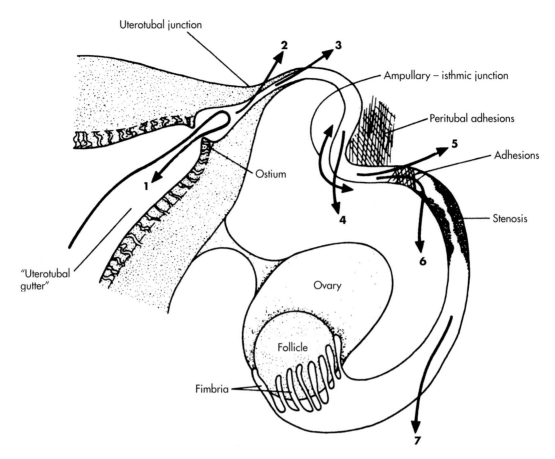

Fig. 13-12. Primary sites at risk for perforation during tubal cannulation before fallosposcopy. (Reprinted with permission from Kerin JF et al: In Corfman RS et al: *Complications of laparoscopy and hysteroscopy,* Boston, 1993, Blackwell Scientific Publications, Fig. 43-1.)

cause of fibrotic obstruction all predispose the fallopian tubes to perforation. No perforations occurring during procedures we have performed have been associated with significant sequelae. A crucial means of avoiding this complication is gentle manipulation and a keen awareness of tubal anatomy.

MANAGEMENT DECISIONS

Proximal disease

Patients with intralumenal mucous plugs or debris may best be managed with aquadissection techniques.[14,16] Intralumenal endometriosis and endosalpingiosis may best be treated medically with a trial of GnRH agonist or danazol therapy, although minimal intralumenal adhesions may be more appropriately approached with gentle guidewire dissection.[1,15,16] Denser adhesions or mild stenoses may also be approached employing balloon dilation techniques.[1,14,16] These procedures could possibly be performed in an office setting once sufficient data addressing safety and patient tolerance have been reported. Increased analgesic requirements and an inability to avoid tubal perforation by performing concomitant laparoscopy may prove to be limiting factors.

Patients with dense fibrotic obstruction require tubal bypass with IVF or resection and microsurgical anastomosis as appropriate.

The patient with suspected hydrosalpinges is managed differently. If a grossly dilated tube with no functional endothelial lining or extensive intralumenal adhesions is noted at falloposcopy, further surgical intervention may prove unnecessary. The patient should be referred directly for IVF. If, however, the lining appears only minimally compromised, laparoscopic assessment of peritubal disease with the potential for neosalpingostomy should be performed. IVF would be appropriate in the face of extensive peritubal disease or more advanced maternal age. This management paradigm is summarized in the box on page 139.

CONCLUSION

Falloposcopy represents an exciting new and evolving technology in which the entire tubal lumen may be visualized with minimum invasion. This procedure clearly lends itself to performance in an office setting with minimal anesthesia. As a result, management decisions can now be made based upon actual visualization of pathologic findings. As experience and technology progress, falloposcopy may be-

Management based on findings at office falloposcopy

Normal lumen

Treat as unexplained infertility
Perform laparoscopy if indicated

Suspected proximal occlusion

Mucous plugs, debris: Aquadissection
Endometriosis, endosalpingiosis: Medical suppression
Nonobstructive adhesions: Guidewire dissection
Moderate adhesions, stenosis: Guidewire dissection or directed balloon tuboplasty
Dense obstruction: IVF/ET vs. resection and microsurgical anastomosis

Suspected distal occlusion

Severe disease: IVF/ET
Mild to moderate disease: IVF/ET vs. laparoscopy, possible neosalpingostomy depending on patient age and extent of peritubal disease

come a standard part of the outpatient evaluation of the infertile patient with suspected tubal disease.

ACKNOWLEDGEMENTS

Special thanks to John F. Kerin, M.D., Ph.D., for his vision, guidance, and pioneering leadership in the development of office falloposcopy and to Ron Arzaga, B.A., for his superb typographic skills.

REFERENCES

1. Kerin J et al: Falloposcopy: a microendoscopic technique for diagnosing and treating endotubal disease incorporating guide wire cannulation and direct balloon tuboplasty, *J Reprod Med* 35:606-12, 1990.
2. Kerin J et al: Falloposcopy: a microendoscopic technique for visual exploration of the human fallopian tube from the uterotubal ostium to the fimbria using a transvaginal approach, *Fertil Steril* 54:390-400, 1990.
3. Sulak P et al: Histology of proximal tubal obstruction. *Fertil Steril* 56:831-5, 1991.
4. Surrey ES, Surrey MW: The role of transfimbrial salpingoscopy in the management of distal tubal disease: correlation with traditional criterion. Abstract P-1 presented at program of the 22nd Annual Meeting of the Pacific Coast Fertility Society, Indian Wells, Calif., April 20-24, 1994.
5. Kerin JF: Nonhysteroscopic falloposcopy: a proposed method for visual guidance and verification of tubal cannula placement for endotuboplasty, gamete, and embryo transfer procedures, *Fertil Steril* 57:1133-5, 1992.
6. Scudamore IW, Dunphy BC, Cooke ID: Outpatient falloposcopy: intralumenal imaging of the fallopian tube by trans-uterine fiber-optic endoscopy as an outpatient procedure, *Br J Obstet Gynecol* 99:829-35, 1992.
7. Venezia R et al: Initial experience of a new linear everting falloposcopy system in comparison with hysterosalpingography, *Fertil Steril* 60:771-5, 1993.
8. Dunphy BC: Office falloposcopy assessment in proximal tubal disease, *Fertil Steril* 61:168-70, 1994.
9. Pearlstone AC, Surrey ES, Kerin JF: The linear everting catheter: a nonhysteroscopic, transvaginal technique for access and microendoscopy of the fallopian tube, *Fertil Steril* 58:854-7, 1992.
10. Bauer O et al: Transcervical access and intra-luminal imaging of the fallopian tube in the nonanesthetized patient: preliminary results using a new technique for fallopian access, *Hum Reprod* 7(Suppl):7-11, 1992.
11. Dunphy B et al: A comparison of pain experienced during hysterosalpingography and in-office falloposcopy, *Fertil Steril* 62:62-70, 1994.
12. Kerin J et al: Falloposcopic classification and treatment of fallopian tube lumen disease, *Fertil Steril* 57:731-41, 1992.
13. Grow DR, Coddington CC, Flood JF: Proximal tubal occlusion by hysterosalpingogram: a role for falloposcopy, *Fertil Steril* 60:170-4, 1993.
14. Kerin JF, Surrey ES: Tubal surgery from the inside out: falloposcopy and balloon tuboplasty. *Clin Obstet Gynecol* 35:299-312, 1992.
15. Kerin JF, Pearlstone AC, Surrey ES: Cannulation of the fallopian tube and falloposcopy: difficulties and complications. In Corfman RS, Diamond MP, DeCherney A, Eds: *Complications of laparoscopy and hysteroscopy,* Boston, 1993, Blackwell Scientific Publications.
16. Kerin J et al: Development and application of a falloposcope for transvaginal endoscopy of the fallopian tube, *J Laparoscopic Surg* 1:47-56, 1990.

Chapter 14

OFFICE ENDOMETRIAL ABLATION

Johnny Awwad

Abnormal uterine bleeding is a frustrating experience in a woman's life and accounts for approximately one third of all gynecologic complaints. Hysterectomy has long been considered the standard surgical approach to this problem. It is estimated that more than 600,000 hysterectomies are performed yearly in the United States, of which 20% to 40% are done for abnormal uterine bleeding.[1,2] A hysterectomy carries an overall mortality rate of 6 per 10,000 and a morbidity rate of 42.8%.[3,4] It is also associated with significant financial burden and considerable physical and emotional stress. With trends in surgical practice favoring more minimally invasive therapy, the management of abnormal uterine bleeding in women has shifted dramatically away from hysterectomy and more toward conservative and directed surgical approaches.

Several minimally invasive surgical alternatives are being investigated to reduce the surgical trauma and risks associated with hysterectomy. These new surgical alternatives have focused on uterine preservation and reduction of abnormal menstrual flow by destroying the regenerative capacity of the endometrium, i.e., endometrial ablation. Currently, acceptable techniques of endometrial ablation include the use of the Nd:YAG laser,[5-7] loop resection,[8] and roller-ball coagulation[9] through an operative hysteroscopic approach under direct visual monitoring. The advantages of endometrial ablation over hysterectomy include a reduced hospital stay, shortened convalescence period, decreased surgical risks, and reduced financial costs. Current hysteroscopic ablation techniques, however, are not without risks and include fluid overload and electrolyte imbalance secondary to the use of large volumes of fluids necessary for uterine distention, the use of potentially hazardous energy sources that can cause accidental injuries,[10] and the requirement of general or regional anesthesia within operating room facilities. In addition, the surgery should only be performed by a highly skilled, experienced surgeon.

Recent research interests have thus focused on further reducing the logistic burdens and potential risks associated with operative hysteroscopy by developing surgical techniques that can ultimately be performed in the office setting. This chapter reviews several office-based techniques to perform endometrial ablation for abnormal uterine bleeding. Although still experimental, many of these therapies possess promising potential and are the result of significant creativity and ingenuity.

NOVEL INVESTIGATIONAL TECHNIQUES OF ENDOMETRIAL ABLATION

The concept of inducing endometrial damage to achieve reduction or complete cessation of bleeding in women with dysfunctional uterine bleeding is not novel. Several successful and unsuccessful attempts have been made in the past to destroy the uterine endometrium with various toxic chemicals and physical agents. The majority of these techniques met with poor success and were associated with significant complications. Examples of several techniques include the use of silver nitrate, fumic nitric acid, quinacrine, urea, cyanoacrylate ester, paraformaldehyde, heated steam, radium packing, and fibroblast implants.[11-16] All of these methods have yielded disappointing results.

Recent investigations have included the use of photodynamic therapy, radiofrequency diathermy, balloon diathermy, and cryosurgery as alternative techniques for endometrial ablation. Whereas hysteroscopy provides direct visualization of the extirpative process, these alternative therapies are blind techniques. In the absence of visual monitoring, the main concern with these procedures lies in the uncertainty of complete endometrial destruction. Theoretically the likelihood of incomplete endometrial destruction, particularly in remote areas of the uterine cavity such as the cornua, could increase. However, the attraction of these novel techniques is their simplicity of use, requiring few surgical skills and precluding the need for operative hysteroscopic manipulation. The procedures potentially can be learned rapidly, resulting in fewer complications and a uniform success rate. Other possible advantages include fewer operative risks because of the absence of uterine fluid distention and significant financial savings because of the reduced need for anesthesia and operating room facilities.

Photodynamic endometrial ablation

The use of lasers in surgical practice has gained wide acceptance. In gynecologic practice the effect of laser energy on tissue is entirely mediated through the photothermal conversion of laser light energy into heat. However, other properties of laser light can be medically useful. Photodynamic therapy, for example, is based on a different laser-tissue interaction. The photodynamic effect is mediated through photochemical destruction of abnormal tissues by activation of photosensitizing compounds on exposure to light of a particular energy and wavelength. Cell death is caused by highly reactive oxygen intermediates generated from the photoactive excitation of molecular oxygen, resulting in irreversible oxidation of vital cellular components.[17-19] To work, photodynamic therapy requires the presence of a photosensitizing compound, oxygen, and light. Cytotoxicity manifests itself in the cytoplasm, mitochondria, and lysosomal membrane with minimal effect on nuclear DNA. Tissue destruction is thought to result either from direct cytotoxic action to the undesirable tissue or damage to its vascular network, resulting in coagulation necrosis.

The principle of selective tissue destruction, wherein normal tissue is spared, using photodynamic therapy requires the preferential localization of an exogenously administered photosensitizing compound within the target tissue. This can be achieved either through increased uptake and/or delayed clearance of the photosensitizing compound within the tissue to be destroyed. Tissue selectivity is primarily a function of tissue vascularity and neovascularization.[20] The excitation wavelength of the laser light is selected to match the absorption band of the photosensitizer for efficient photoactivation. Overlap with the absorption spectrum of endogenous tissue pigments such as hemoglobin and melanin can impair adequate tissue penetration.

Photodynamic therapy has been applied to treat various malignant and benign diseases.[21-27] Its application to the endometrial cavity to manage dysfunctional uterine bleeding is relatively novel. By virtue of its prominent vascularity, the endometrium has the potential to sequester and retain photosensitizing compounds in a preferential fashion compared with surrounding tissues.[28] The uterine cavity, by being a well-confined space naturally protected by the thick myometrium, represents an ideal site in which to apply the photodynamic effect. Because of the limited depth of light penetration through the myometrium, activation of the photosensitizer past the endometrium is unlikely. The myometrium provides a natural protection for adjacent intra-abdominal organs.

Animal data[28-31] suggest that photodynamic therapy is an effective approach for selective endometrial destruction. Bhatta et al[28] demonstrated that photofrin, a photosensitizing compound, is taken up and retained preferentially by rabbit endometrium 24 hours following administration. When the photofrin was activated by laser light within the rabbit uterine horns, there was complete nonthermal necrosis of the endometrium, partial destruction of the myometrium, and sparing of the serosa. Yang et al[30] demonstrated a long-lasting photodynamic effect on rat endometrium in vivo using topically applied 5-aminolevulinic acid. Photodynamic ablation using this photosensitizer resulted in destruction of the rat endometrium and persistent disruption of endometrial function despite strong hormonal stimulation. The reproductive capability of the uterine horns was profoundly affected as long as 60 days after treatment as demonstrated by a reduction in the implantation rate from 100% to 16.7%.[30] Similar results were obtained in both rats and rabbits by Wyss et al[32] using the same methodology.

In view of the experimental success of photodynamic endometrial ablation in animal models,[28-32] it has become evident that the procedure can have significant therapeutic potential in women with abnormal uterine bleeding. A clinical trial is under way at Massachusetts General Hospital to evaluate the efficacy and safety of this approach. The success of this minimally invasive approach is dependent upon several factors among which are the optical and pharmacokinetic properties of the photosensitizing agent, its mode of administration, light dosimetry, and timing of light therapy. The technique can be summarized by the administration of a photosensitizing compound followed by endometrial irradiation, using a low-power light of a particular wavelength generated by an argon-pumped dye laser (Fig. 14-1). The intrauterine light delivery system consists of a balloon device that allows homogenous light distribution and equal spatial light delivery upon inflation inside the uterine cavity.

Most of the clinical data reported to date with photodynamic therapy are derived from the use of hematoporphyrin derivatives and photofrin. These photosensitizing agents have been shown to have a destructive effect on tumor microvasculature and hence are highly effective in well-vascularized tissues.[33,34] They are photoactivated by red light at a wavelength of 630 nm. Prolonged retention, however, has been shown in several organs and has been reported to persist up to 4 to 6 weeks. During this period, patients are highly photosensitive, and exposure to sun or bright indoor lights can result in serious skin burns.[35] Special filters to shield operating room lights are also required to prevent activation of the photosensitizer in intra-abdominal organs should a surgical procedure be necessary during the period of photosensitivity.

Because the length of the photosensitivity period is a function of the pharmacokinetic properties of the compound

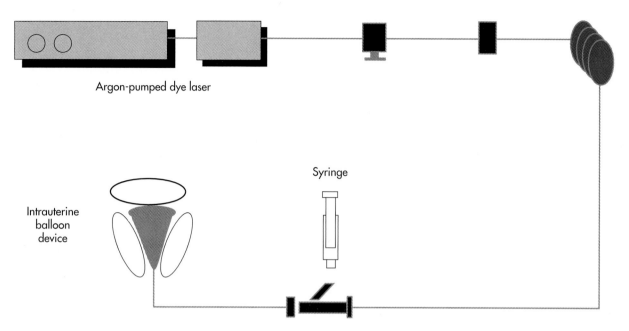

Fig. 14-1. Photodynamic therapy for endometrial ablation. Light from an argon-pumped dye laser is delivered to the endometrium through an intrauterine balloon device, causing photoactivation of the photosensitizing compound.

used, a newer generation of photosensitizers has recently been developed to circumvent the potential serious side effects of photosensitivity. These compounds can improve treatment efficacy while reducing the period of tissue retention. Phthalocyanines, chlorins, 5-aminolevulinic acid, and benzoporphyrin derivatives have been demonstrated to possess promising photodynamic effects with reduced cutaneous toxicity.[18] 5-aminolevulinic acid is a precursor of protoporphyrin IX, a potent photosensitizer. Because conversion of the latter into heme occurs slowly, administration of exogenous 5-aminolevulinic acid induces accumulation of protoporphyrin IX.[36] The photosensitivity period associated with 5-aminolevulinic acid administration is short, not exceeding a few days. Moreover, protoporphyrin IX conversion from 5-aminolevulinic acid is tissue specific and occurs preferentially in the endometrium rather than the myometrium.

Topical intrauterine delivery of photosensitizing compounds has been suggested as another method of reducing the side effects associated with systemic administration. This site-specific delivery has been shown to provide a higher local concentration of the drug with minimal systemic absorption in animal models. Endometrial fluorescence following intrauterine photofrin administration has demonstrated significantly higher concentrations of endometrial photofrin than both the intravenous and intraperitoneal routes.[31] A ten-fold reduction in drug dose was achieved with the intrauterine route for comparable tissue fluorescence. Nevertheless, the practical considerations related to the applicability of this mode of drug delivery to the human endometrium are more complex. The use of high-

viscosity carrier media is required to maximize retention of the photosensitizer inside the uterine cavity. Uniform and homogenous distribution of the drug over the entire endometrial surface remains a concern in view of retrograde regurgitation through the cervix and spillage through the fallopian tubes. The risk of infection caused by repeated and prolonged intrauterine manipulations is also a concern.

The chief criticism of photodynamic therapy for endometrial ablation is the limited availability and costliness of laser equipment. This equipment is currently space-occupying and difficult to operate and requires high maintenance. For these reasons, there recently has been a growing interest in developing a newer generation of laser sources that can meet the requirements for office use, i.e., that the laser sources be affordable, mobile, compact, and self-sustainable, and require low maintenance. Because photodynamic therapy requires a low-power light energy, diode lasers are good candidates and show strong promise for this task.

Acceptance of photodynamic endometrial ablation to manage dysfunctional uterine bleeding in women depends largely on the development of new photosensitizers with limited phototoxicity and on the availability of affordable laser systems designed for office use.

Radiofrequency ablation

The use of radiofrequency electromagnetic energy to produce diathermy in body cavities is not new.[37] This approach has been described for the treatment of a variety of benign and malignant conditions such as benign prostatic hyperplasia,[38,39] carcinoma of the cervix,[40] and various gas-

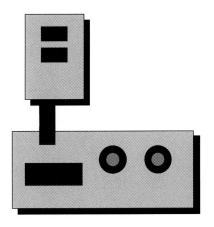

"Menostat" radiofrequency ablation unit

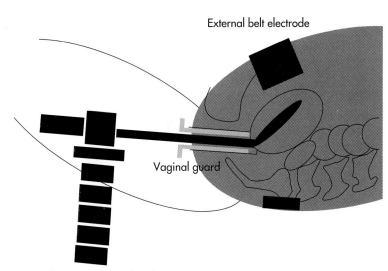

Radiofrequency thermal probe

Fig. 14-2. Radiofrequency endometrial ablation. A high-frequency signal is applied to the radiofrequency thermal probe, causing energy to be deposited in the endometrium in the form of heat. An insulated vaginal guard is used to protect the bladder and rectum.

trointestinal conditions.[41] However, the use of radiofrequency ablation to induce irreversible thermal damage to the endometrium as an alternative surgical approach to dysfunctional uterine bleeding is new.[42]

The technique consists of placing a 10-mm-diameter, stainless steel conductive probe into the uterine cavity (Fig. 14-2). An insulated belt electrode around the patient's waist acts as a ground electrode. A high-frequency signal (27.12 MHz) with an incident power of 550 W and an energy dose of 330 to 660 kJ is applied to the radiofrequency thermal probe, depositing energy into the endometrium in the form of heat. Because radiofrequency hyperthermia results from capacitative coupling between the probe and the endometrial tissue, the irregularity of the endometrial cavity does not preclude whole-cavity heating. The system is designed such that the surface of the probe is significantly smaller than the return electrode. As a result, the electric field strength drops inversely with the distance from the probe, limiting the thermal effect to the endometrium and the inner layers of the myometrium. Thermometry studies on treated uteri revealed an intracavitary temperature of 60° to 65° C at the endometrial surface, 50° to 57° C at a depth of 5 mm, and no temperature change at the serosal surface of the uterus.[42,43]

Earlier experience with this technique revealed that 30% of patients treated achieved a reduction in menstrual flow.[44] Following appropriate modifications of the energy dose and the radiofrequency probe design, Phipps et al[42] subsequently treated 33 patients with menorrhagia and reported an overall success rate of 85%. Amenorrhea was achieved in 30% of patients and reduction of blood flow in 55%. Some patients required repeat procedures. A 74% reduction in blood loss[45] was demonstrated in 15 patients using the radioactive ^{59}Fe

iron/whole body gamma counting method.[46] No evidence of deleterious systemic effects were noted as a result of heat-altered blood draining from the uterus, as demonstrated by the absence of red-cell deformity or alteration in coagulation profile.

A blood-stained vaginal discharge was reported by most patients for 1 to 4 weeks following the procedure. Serious complications can result from the patient coming in contact with a conducting object that will attract a flow of current and result in an unintentional burn. Hence any metallic surface that is in close contact with the patient, such as the stirrup pole frames, operating room table frame, and pulse oximeter probe, can cause severe burns to the patient. Skin burns have indeed been reported at the site of ECG electrodes, requiring the placement of special filters between the leads and monitor.[45,47] Accidental injury to the anterior vaginal wall also occurred in two patients, resulting in vesicovaginal fistulas. An insulated thermal guard now must be used in the vagina to protect the bladder and rectum. It is imperative that the surgeon and assisting staff be sharply aware of the guidelines for safe practice and that these guidelines be followed rigorously.

Thermal balloon ablation

The use of diathermy through heated steam to destroy the endometrial lining has been reported in medical literature. This practice, however, has produced severe intraperitoneal burns, resulting in patient fatalities.[48] A modified approach has recently been described using a newly designed balloon device to deliver the thermal energy in a more controlled and safe fashion.[49,50]

The balloon thermal ablation system consists of a latex balloon that is filled with a solution of 5% dextrose in water

(Fig. 14-3). The balloon contains a shielded heating element that is activated to heat the liquid in the balloon to 92° C by convection currents. The temperature is set just below the boiling point of the fluid to prevent steam formation and pressure build-up inside the balloon. The catheter is connected to a control panel that regulates time, temperature, and pressure. The system is designed to recognize uterine perforation or balloon rupture by shutting down when the intrauterine pressure falls acutely. Safety and efficacy studies performed on the thermal balloon device[50] showed a uniform coagulation depth of 3 to 5 mm into the endometrium with no significant temperature changes at the serosal surface of the uterus.

Singer et al[49] described the treatment of 18 women with menorrhagia by the thermal balloon technique. This approach resulted in significant reduction or total elimination of menstrual bleeding in 83% of patients over a 6- to 34-month follow-up. Both histopathology and postoperative hysteroscopy of treated uteri supported thermal burn with scar formation as the mechanism of endometrial destruction.

Multielectrode balloon endometrial ablation

The VestaBlate System* is a novel approach for blind endometrial ablation.[51] It consists of a multielectrode, conformable balloon that delivers electrical power in the form of heat to the endometrial lining. A controller unit regulates energy to each of the balloon electrodes via temperature sensors. The electrode balloon is introduced into the uterine cavity through an inserter and is then inflated with air, allowing intimate contact between the electrodes and endometrium. A 4-minute therapeutic phase is required for a complete therapeutic effect. During that time, the en-

*Vesta Medical, Mountain View, Calif.

dometrium is heated to 70° to 75° C. Initial in vivo prehysterectomy studies performed on 30 women revealed the absence of significant serosal temperature build-up. The depth of necrosis into the myometrium averaged 2 to 4 mm. Clinical data evaluating efficacy and safety are not yet available.

Cryosurgery

Conflicting data exist in medical literature about the success of cryosurgery to treat dysfunctional uterine bleeding.[52-56] Cahan and Brockunier[52] treated six patients with abnormal uterine bleeding using intrauterine applications of circulating liquid nitrogen at −80° C. One patient developed complete amenorrhea; four others had normalization of their periods, and one failed therapy. A single patient developed pelvic abscesses following the procedure. Subsequent experience with the use of Freon as the cooling agent was unsatisfactory.[53] Using this technique, Droegemueller, Greer, and Makowski[54] treated 16 patients with functional menorrhagia with a single freeze-thaw cycle at −40° C. Incomplete endometrial destruction and sparing of both cornual ends was observed in all patients. It was soon recognized that the limitation associated with Freon use was related to its high boiling point. Nitrous oxide was then used by the same investigators as an alternative cooling agent in 11 patients, using a single freeze-thaw cycle at intracavitary temperatures of −60° C. All patients underwent a hysterectomy 6 to 8 weeks following treatment.[55] Upon gross examination of the uteri, the anterior and posterior uterine walls were found to be in direct apposition. Coagulation necrosis with or without hyalinization was the most common histologic finding, extending to approximately 25% of the myometrial thickness. Complete ablation was observed in three patients and partial ablation in the remaining eight patients with skip areas in the cornua and fundus.

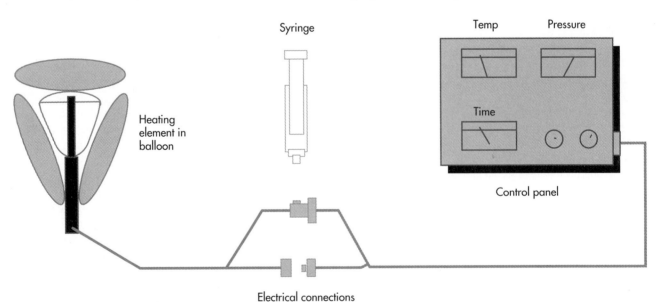

Fig. 14-3. Thermal balloon endometrial ablation. Heating elements serve to heat the liquid inside the balloon, resulting in thermal effect to the endometrium.

Endometrial cryosurgery results in coagulation necrosis caused by subfreezing temperatures. Cell death is caused by physical rupture of cell walls with intracellular and extracellular ice crystal formation and avascular necrosis produced by vascular thrombosis. The safety of cryosurgery has been demonstrated following in vivo and in vitro intracavitary treatment studies of the uterus, in which no significant drop in temperature was detected at the serosal surface during congelation.[52]

The interpretation of clinical data on endometrial cryosurgery is ambiguous, mostly because of the paucity of available studies and the absence of a uniform method of cryotherapy. For this reason, the value of cryosurgery for endometrial ablation in women with dysfunctional uterine bleeding remains to be determined.

Hysteroscopic endometrial ablation under local anesthesia

With instrumental technology unfolding rapidly, more surgical techniques previously performed in a standard operative setting now have the potential of becoming office procedures. Diagnostic hysteroscopy is the perfect example, and operative hysteroscopy as well is no exception.

Recently Hill, Maher, and Lloyd[57] recommended using local anesthesia for operative hysteroscopy. They performed hysteroscopic endometrial ablations on 20 patients, using intravenous midazolam and fentanyl for sedation and paracervical and uterosacral infiltration with a mixture of bupivacaine and lidocaine for local anesthesia. The "rollerball" technique was used for endometrial electrocoagulation, using glycine for uterine distention. All patients tolerated the procedure well. Twelve patients reported momentary discomfort upon ablation of the tubal ostia. Nineteen patients admitted satisfaction from the anesthetic technique, expressing willingness to use it in the future if necessary.

Because early symptoms of glycine toxicity and uterine perforation are most easily recognized when the patient is awake, the use of local anesthesia may be more advantageous than general anesthesia for quick detection of these complications. Shortened postoperative recovery is another advantage associated with local anesthesia. This technique nevertheless relies heavily on the attitude of the patient and her willingness to cooperate throughout the procedure. With increasing financial pressures, it will only be a matter of time before additional similar trials will be performed.

FUTURE PERSPECTIVES

With growing interest in minimally invasive surgery, the list of hysterectomy alternatives to treat dysfunctional uterine bleeding is constantly expanding. The potential benefits of the new techniques are enormous. Among the benefits are reduced surgical and anesthetic risks, shortened recovery time, and improved patient convenience. Capital costs of equipment can be rapidly offset by savings gained from the reduced need for operating room time and professional staff, absence

of hospitalization, and decreased convalescence period. Because these novel investigational techniques in practice do not require advanced surgical skills, they can be performed by well-trained technicians, thereby opening the procedures to a greater number of health care providers. For this reason, these procedures are ideal for use in physician-deficient developing countries, where medical needs and demands far outweigh the number of professional health care providers and the availability of surgical facilities. The use of these novel techniques for endometrial ablation may also represent a valuable alternative to operative hysteroscopy in a well-selected subgroup of women who are medically compromised and at high risk for general anesthesia and fluid overload.

The potential complications associated with the use of these novel techniques are still unknown. Long-term studies and cumulative experience will reveal their safety and success and ultimately determine their acceptability. Controversy is an essential component of any novelty. Yet it is through continuous criticism that these novel techniques will attain ultimate refinement and will better accommodate health care needs. The effect of such minimally invasive therapy could be dramatic as it may influence the core content of operative gynecology. Nevertheless, it is equally important that these revolutionary procedures be properly assessed before being introduced for general use.

REFERENCES

1. Easterday CL, Grimes DA, Riggs JA: Hysterectomy in the United States, *Obstet Gynecol* 62:203, 1983.
2. Pokras R, Hufnagel VG: Hysterectomies in the United States 1965-1984. DHHS publication No. (PHS) 87-1753. Vital and health statistics, series 13; No. 92, 1-32. Hyattsville, Maryland, 1987, Centers for Disease Control, National Center for Health Statistics.
3. Wingo PA et al: The mortality risk associated with hysterectomy, *Am J Obstet Gynecol* 152:803, 1985.
4. Dicker RC et al: Complications of abdominal and vaginal hysterectomy among women of reproductive age in the United States, *Am J Obstet Gynecol* 144:841, 1982.
5. Goldrath MH, Fuller T, Segal S: Laser photovaporization of endometrium for the treatment of menorrhagia, *Am J Obstet Gynecol* 140:14, 1981.
6. Lomano JM: Photocoagulation of the endometrium with the Nd-YAG laser for the treatment of menorrhagia, *J Reprod Med* 31:148, 1986.
7. Loffer FD: Hysteroscopic endometrial ablation with the Nd-YAG laser using a nontouch technique, *Obstet Gynecol* 69:679, 1987.
8. DeCherney A, Polan ML: Hysteroscopic management of intrauterine lesions and intractable uterine bleeding, *Obstet Gynecol* 61:392, 1983.
9. Vancaillie TG: Electrocoagulation of the endometrium with the ball-end resectoscope, *Obstet Gynecol* 74:425, 1981.
10. MacDonald R, Phipps J, Singer A: Endometrial ablation: a safe procedure, *Gynaecol Endosc* 1:7, 1992.
11. Crossen RJ, Crossen HS: Radiation therapy of uterine myoma, *JAMA* 133:593, 1947.
12. Rongy AJ: Radium therapy in benign uterine bleeding, *J of the Mount Sinai Hosp* 14:569, 1947.
13. Polishuk WZ, Schenker JG: Induction of intrauterine adhesions in the rabbit with autologous fibroblast implants, *Am J Obstet Gynecol* 115:789, 1973.
14. Schenker JG et al: An in vitro fibroblast-enriched sponge preparation for induction of intrauterine adhesions, *Isr J Med Sci* 11:849, 1975.

15. Tilt EJ: *A handbook of uterine therapeutics: caustic medication,* ed 4, New York, 1881, William Wood.

16. Goldrath MH: In Sharp F and Jordan JA, Eds: *Gynaecological laser surgery: hysteroscopic laser ablation of the endometrium,* New York, 1987, Publishers Perinatology Press.

17. Weishaupt KR, Gomer CJ, Dougherty TJ: Identification of singlet oxygen as the cytotoxic agent in photoinactivation of a murine tumor, *Cancer Res* 36:2326, 1976.

18. Kimel S et al: Singlet oxygen generation of porphyrins, chlorins, and phthalocyanines, *Photochem Photobiol* 50:175, 1989.

19. Kreimer-Birnbaum M: Modified porphyrins, chlorins, phthalocyanines, and purpurines: second generation photosensitizers for photodynamic therapy, *Semin Hematol* 26:157, 1989.

20. Roberts WG, Hassan T: Role of neovasculature and vascular permeability on the tumor retention of photodynamic agents, *Cancer Res* 52:924, 1992.

21. Dougherty TJ et al: Photoradiation in the treatment of recurrent breast carcinoma, *J Natl Cancer Inst* 62:231, 1979.

22. Benson RC: Laser photodynamic therapy for bladder cancer, *Mayo Clin Proc* 61:859, 1986.

23. Edell ES, Cortese DA: Bronchoscopic phototherapy with hematoporphyrin derivative for treatment of localized bronchogenic carcinoma: a 5-year experience, *Mayo Clin Proc* 62:8, 1987.

24. McCaughan JS et al: Palliation of esophageal malignancy with photoradiation therapy, *Cancer* 54:2905, 1984.

25. DeLaney TF et al: Phase I study of debulking surgery and photodynamic therapy for disseminated intraperitoneal tumors, *Int J Radiat Oncol Biol Phys* 25:445, 1993.

26. Soma H et al: Treatment of vaginal carcinoma with laser photoirradiation following administration of hematoporphyrin derivative, *Ann Chir Gynaecol* 71:133, 1982.

27. Rettenmaier MA et al: Photoradiation therapy of gynecologic malignancies, *Gynecol Oncol* 17:200, 1984.

28. Bhatta N et al: Endometrial ablation by means of photodynamic therapy with photofrin II, *Am J Obstet Gynecol* 167:1856, 1992.

29. Schneider D et al: Endometrial ablation by DHE photoradiation therapy in estrogen treated ovariectomized rats, *Colposc Gynecol Laser Surg* 4:73, 1988.

30. Yang JZ et al: Evidence of lasting functional destruction of the rat endometrium after 5-aminolevulinic acid-induced photodynamic ablation: prevention of implantation, *Am J Obstet Gynecol* 168:995, 1993.

31. Chapman JA et al: Effect of administration route and estrogen manipulation on endometrial uptake of photofrin, *Am J Obstet Gynecol* 168:685, 1993.

32. Wyss P et al: Photodynamic destruction of endometrial tissue with topical 5-aminolevulinic acid in rats and rabbits, *Am J Obstet Gynecol* 171:1176, 1994.

33. Lipson RL, Baldes EJ, Gray MJ: Hematoporphyrin derivative for detection and management of cancer, *Cancer* 20:2255, 1967.

34. Star WM et al: Destruction of rat mammary tumor and normal tissue microcirculation by hematoporphyrin derivative photoradiation observed in vivo in sandwich observation chambers, *Cancer Res* 46:2532, 1986.

35. Kennedy JC, Pottier RH, Pross DC: Photodynamic therapy with endogenous protopophyrin IX: basic principles and present clinical experience, *Photochem Photobiol* 6:143, 1990.

36. Kennedy JC, Pottier RH: Endogeneous protoporphyrin IX, a clinically useful photosensitizer for photodynamic therapy, *J Photochem Photobiol* 14:275, 1992.

37. Schliephake E: *Short wave therapy,* London, 1935, Actinic Press.

38. Yerushalmi A et al: Localized deep microwave hyperthermia in the treatment of poor operative risk patients with benign prostatic hyperplasia, *J Urology* 133:873, 1985.

39. Astrahan MA et al: Microwave applicator for transurethral hyperthermia of benign prostatic hyperplasia, *Int J Hyperthermia* 5:283, 1989.

40. Hand JW et al: *Clinical Thermobiology: a coaxial applicator for intracavitary hyperthermia of carcinoma of the cervix,* Gautherie M and Albert E, New York, 1982, Alan R Liss.

41. Oliguchi Y, Tsutsumi S: *Hyperthermic oncology: RF capacitative heating by electrode inserted in stomach and outer one,* vol 1, Sugahara M and Saito M, London, 1989, Taylor & Francis.

42. Phipps JH et al: Experimental and clinical studies with radiofrequency-induced thermal endometrial ablation for functional menorrhagia, *Obstet Gynecol* 76:876, 1990.

43. Prior MV et al: Treatment of menorrhagia by radiofrequency heating, *Int J Hyperthermia* 7:213, 1991.

44. Phipps JH et al: Treatment of functional menorrhagia by radiofrequency induced thermal endometrial ablation, *Lancet* 335(i):374, 1990.

45. Phipps JH, Lewis BV: *Endoscopic surgery for gynaecologists: radiofrequency endometrial ablation (RaFEA).* In Sutton C and Diamond M, Eds: *Endoscopic Surgery for Gynaecologists,* London, 1993, WB Saunders.

46. Holt JM et al: Measurement of blood loss by means of a whole body counter, *BMJ* 4:86, 1967.

47. Page VJ: Anaesthesia and radiofrequency endometrial ablation, *Eur J Anaesthesiol* 10:25, 1993.

48. Hardt W, Genz T: Atmokausis—Vaporisation. Schwerste innere Verbrennungen nach intrauteriner Anwendung von Strömenden Wasserdampf, *Geburtshilfe Frauenheilkd* 49:293, 1989.

49. Singer A et al: Preliminary clinical experience with a thermal balloon endometrial ablation method to treat menorrhagia, *Obstet Gynecol* 83:732, 1994.

50. Neuwirth RS et al: The endometrial ablator: a new instrument, *Obstet Gynecol* 83:792, 1994.

51. Vancaillie TG, Stern RA: A novel multi-electrode balloon for endometrial ablation, *Contemp Obstet Gynecol* Apr 15:44, 1995.

52. Cahan WG, Brockunier A: Cryosurgery of the uterine cavity, *Am J Obstet Gynecol* 99:138, 1967.

53. Droegemueller W, Greer BE, Makowski EL: *Am J Obstet Gynecol* 107:958, 1970.

54. Droegemueller W, Greer B, Makowski E: Cryosurgery in patients with dysfunctional uterine bleeding, *Obstet Gynecol* 38:256, 1971.

55. Droegemueller W, Malowski E, Macsulka R: Destruction of the endometrium by cryosurgery, *Am J Obstet Gynecol* 110:467, 1971.

56. Droegemueller W et al: Cryocoagulation of the endometrium at the uterine cornua, *Am J Obstet Gynecol* 131:1, 1978.

57. Hill DJ, Maher PJ, Lloyd D: Endometrial ablation under local analgesia, *Aust N Z J Obstet Gynaecol* 32:284, 1992.

INDEX